CAMBODIA
2000
The AIDS Year

MARGARET ATKIN

Published by Margaret Atkin

Licensed under Creative Commons BY-NC license.

Contact margaretatkin.com on Facebook

https://www.facebook.com/margaretatkinauthor

creative commons license CC BY-NC 4.0

Attribution-Noncommercial

4.00 International

First published in Australia 2025

Copyright © Margaret Atkin 2025

Cover design, typesetting: WorkingType (www.workingtype.com.au)

Cover image: Margaret and young girl in Thma Puok near Thai border.

Margaret Atkin

Cambodia 2000 – The AIDS Year

ISBN: 9780646712574

To my Khmer and Australian families, and work colleagues during the epidemic in 2000 and 2001; and to those with HIV, their families, friends and supporting services, who continue to battle this virus in the Asia Pacific region.

margaretatkin.com

CONTENTS

After watching my sister Sue die at 41 from melanoma, my own life felt meaningless. It was August 1998. At her deathbed, with my parents Gill and Ray, and my younger sister Lil, I sensed a powerful presence — one beyond words. I also felt the presence of my brother Pete and his wife Wendy, who had died in a car accident over ten years earlier, along with two of their three children.

Grief consumed me. Night after night, I stood at my window, staring at the darkened park, waiting for dawn. Sleep was elusive. Then, one night, I woke from a vivid dream.

I saw six Asian village women, their faces weathered by the sun, standing in the shade by a dried riverbank. They wore long cotton skirts and called to me, desperate and afraid. Their husbands were dying. If they refused them sex, they were beaten.

I woke knowing I had to find them.

Dreams like this had come before, and they were always right. I began searching for volunteer roles and found an opening with Australian Volunteers International in Cambodia, a country in the grips of the fastest-growing AIDS epidemic in Asia. I had worked as a nurse and journalist in the Solomon Islands, confronting difficult realities before, but this felt different.

I applied, was accepted, and threw myself into learning

everything I could about HIV/AIDS in Cambodia. It was a crisis - one threatening to overwhelm the health system and economy, a silent devastation spreading through brothels and into families. Around a third of Cambodia's brothel-based sex workers tested positive for HIV, and a staggering 60% of Cambodian men admitted to regularly visiting brothels. The women in my dream were right. HIV was moving into the general population, with an infection rate of 3 to 4%. By the previous year, 160,000 people were living with HIV, including 2,200 children. Over 5,000 AIDS orphans had already been left behind.

The weeklong orientation in Melbourne was sobering. A fellow volunteer, a doctor, bluntly told me he wouldn't take such a position. "There are no working hospitals, few labs, and no antiretrovirals," he said. "What can you do?"

He was right. But I went anyway.

When I arrived in Phnom Penh in March 2000, I met Dr Tia Phalla, the man leading Cambodia's fight against AIDS. In 1991, he had recognised that the epidemic had the power to destroy his country, just as Pol Pot had. He formed the National AIDS Committee, travelled across Cambodia, and convinced leaders to act. As Secretary General of the National AIDS Authority, he asked me to go to Poipet, where the crisis was spreading faster than anywhere else.

"They think it's heaven, but it's hell," he said.

I had little confidence, but I would try.

That was over twenty years ago. So why does this story matter now?

Because in February 2025, Fiji and Papua New Guinea are both facing HIV crises - among the worst in the world after Eastern and Southern Africa.

In 2011, Fiji's President Ratu Epeli Nailatikau warned that HIV/AIDS was a ticking time bomb. He called for funding to ensure universal access to treatment and prevention. That didn't happen. Now, the epidemic has exploded, fuelled by injecting drug use and deep-seated stigma. In 2024 alone, over 1,093 new cases were recorded, and half of those living with HIV and aware of their status are not on treatment. UNAIDS has called for urgent, non-discriminatory intervention, backed by Fiji's Minister of Health, Dr Ratu Lalabalavu. Treatment saves lives - but it also stops the virus from spreading. Measures advocated by UNAIDS include Pre-exposure treatment, or treatment taken by an HIV negative person to reduce risk of getting HIV if they are exposed, and needle exchange syringe programs.

In Papua New Guinea, the HIV prevalence rate has reached 1% - the highest in 12 years. In 2024, UN AIDS Regional Director Eamonn Murphy recommended scaling up testing, including self and community-based screening. Pre-exposure therapy, already used in other countries, must become widely available. UNICEF has also urged increased testing for pregnant women, as a third of HIV-positive mothers in PNG are passing the virus to their babies.

The Solomon Islands, too, has seen HIV transmission rise. Between September 2023 and December 2024, seven new cases were recorded - most linked to injecting drug use and men having sex with men. By January 2025, two additional cases were suspected, including a 14-year-old girl diagnosed in hospital.

Dr Jackson Rakei, Director of the Solomon Islands HIV program, has called for an awareness campaign targeting high-risk groups. Deputy Secretary for Health, Dr Nemia Bainivalu, stressed the need for provincial-scale testing and treatment. There is a concern that logging companies operating in remote areas could introduce the virus into rural communities. In 2015 UNAIDS recognised this risk in its report about the HIV/AIDS response in the Solomon Islands.

Dr Rakei is right: addressing HIV requires full community mobilisation and support at every level. That was how we turned the epidemic around in Cambodia in 2000 - without antiretrovirals. Cambodia was one of just three countries in the world that year to successfully reverse the spread of HIV.

The root causes of HIV epidemics - poverty, stigma, and social upheaval - remain. But the fundamental principles of engagement and mobilisation that worked in Cambodia still hold the key today.

Cambodia is no longer the deeply stricken country I entered in 2000. This, then, is the story of our journey.

Chapter One

ORIENTATION PHNOM PENH – MARCH 2000

It was right to come, I thought as I gazed down at the small brown triangular fields and oxen while the plane circled down into Phnom Penh on the second Sunday of March 2000.

I was surprised by that certainty, but it disappeared during the minibus ride into the city. There were four wide lanes with a few land-cruisers and cars, a sea of motorbikes eddying around them. Nobody wore helmets, there were multiple streams of traffic, and everybody ignored the red lights. Motorbikes carried families, live pigs and chickens, while others towed heavy trailers laden with pipes and bricks. There was much beeping of horns. Were there rules, invisible to me as a Westerner, or were the drivers visually challenged psychopaths as my 1996 edition of the Lonely Planet advised.

After being dropped at my hotel and checking the small windowless mould-smelling room, I decided the streets were healthier. I didn't want to lose my nerve. I needed to face that traffic and cross a road. I waited on the sidewalk and studied other pedestrians' techniques. They crossed in groups, a group being harder to mow down. I walked until I found others waiting and crossed. Having made it to the opposite side I looked up. What an extraordinary tangle of wires there was. It looked like each householder attached themselves to the grid, surely at considerable risk. On top of the rooves were little shacks and washing hanging from window poles.

I poked around in the tiny caverns of shops and found everything from old tyres to IV antibiotics, from Valium to pickles. Outside the traffic was quietening, and shops were shutting. It was eleven thirty, time for lunch. Many of the food vendors shut too and gathering in groups played cards. The rickshaw drivers pulled up under the trees and slept in their cabs. Then on the stroke of two it all started again.

I passed one person I still remember. He was a thin, tall, greying man and he spat out, "Animal," as I passed. There was so much hatred in his eyes. I didn't let it trouble me then, but I realise now I probably represented the white people who sent over the b 52 bombers. American bombs, 500,000 tonnes of them, were dropped between 1969 and 1973 to disrupt the supply route to the Viet Cong. They killed hundreds of thousands of Cambodians and were a major factor in the rise of Pol Pot.

By three o'clock I was hungry and managed to buy three mangoes and a couple of bananas by pointing at them. The woman was happy with the note I handed her and gave me some very battered notes as change. Back in my cave I ate the fruit and realised I hadn't brought a book. How stupid! I was an avid reader, and it might be hard to find them here.

At the hotel I met another volunteer, a square short armed

bloke, with a face like Zeus. He made prosthetics. Cambodia had the highest prevalence rate of amputation in the world, 1 per 236 people. I was later told by an expatriate engineer that poor villagers desperate for crops used kitchen knives to clear 90% of the land initially. The worst year was 1996 when 4,320 people were killed or injured but by 1998 it had dropped to 727. The Ministry of Planning in 1999 estimated there were still 4 to 6 million landmines in the ground.

In the evening, I met a volunteer couple and together we went out to eat. We settled on noodles but rinsed the utensils with hot water beforehand to kill any lurking viruses. By seven fifteen it was dark, and we left for the hotel. I hoped the rest of the week would be like this. A holiday I thought wistfully, before facing the awful realities of the job.

The next morning, I was up early to continue my education. Although it was just six the streets were busy. I hadn't realised the hotel was so close to the royal palace until I walked past. It was partially covered with gold leaf, while great rusty chains encircled the closed gates. Opposite the palace a jumble of boys lay sleeping on a tarp. Meanwhile an army of women with twig brooms swept rubbish into heaps, gutters and out of the way places. Judging from the amount of rubbish already there, it had been swept there many times before. Later I saw men collecting it in steel bins and lifting them into a truck with a grinder. Still at least there were jobs, however poorly paid.

Street vendors emerged and set up petrol and kerosene stalls, while an occasional European jogger passed me. In a fun park boys jogged around aging roundabouts and Ferris wheels with one boy painfully thin. Boys, just four or five years old, also very thin, looked for food scraps in receptacles and on the ground at the riverfront.

Chinese music cracked and imperious, grew louder as thirty older people practiced tai chi. Behind them was the Mekong River, junk sails outlined against the first pink crack in a grey dawn. I watched two boys chasing a soccer ball, jump over a wall and run down the steep concrete verge to the river. One slipped into the dirty water while the other laughed. Recovering he swam out, grabbed the ball, and threw it back to his friend. A wave of homesickness overwhelmed me. How could I leave my two teenage sons like I had? What was I thinking of? Then I passed dozens of small birds, each in a single tiny cage. No one had the money or goodwill to free them. I bought a Phnom Penh Post and paid the vendor $A1. She said "ja." It was the first Khmer word I'd understood.

Over breakfast I read the paper. Desperate children and families were scrounging in dumps, pricked by needles, run over by bulldozers, and poisoned by toxins including dioxin. By setting fire to their rubbish dumps the authorities generated very high levels of dioxin which could cause cancer and liver damage. What a country!

At the orientation course the language and history lessons were unexciting and on Tuesday afternoon I was happy to be called away. Riding pillion I was taken to the airport to collect my excess luggage. My role was unclear before I left, and I had brought nurse education books and HIV/AIDS material. I thought I would be working in the nursing school at Battambang and

4

knew as a nurse educator in the Solomons I couldn't rely on local supplies.

Retrieving this excess baggage was my first experience of the unending corruption I was to encounter. First, I had to get the Chief Customs Officer's signature. That cost $A10, and we were told to report back. We got signatures from custom officers with desks under trees who were kicking a shuttle around. One threw a bottle over his shoulder to join the big heap of rubbish already lying there. We peered into a shed where all the air freight for Cambodia was stored, and I watched as a small man sifted through it and found mine. I paid him too. When we reported back to the Chief Customs Officer, he demanded a further $A25. I was lucky it was not more. A woman auditor wanted money too, but my minder turned her down.

Back at the hotel, room service provided an awful meal with uncooked onions, uncooked cabbage, and uncooked beans. The tea had condensed milk in it. I ate one Weetabix afterwards as a treat.

On Wednesday morning I woke after sleeping right through the night. I was settled, but a lunch time visit to the Tuol Sleng Museum changed that. It was a grim cracked concrete building three to four storeys high with the floors divided into cells. In each cell there was a rusty bed, and torture stakes on the floor. There were pictures of swollen blackened corpses on the beds, taken by the Vietnamese when they liberated Phnom Penh in 1979. Twenty thousand people passed through here. On the walls there were photos of young women with babies, young girls, intellectuals, working men, old peasants, and children. Most people looked grim, but one bearded European man was standing, uncowed. There was another of a young boy standing amongst a sea of sleeping people. There were many photos of people taken side on, an arrow pointing to the back of their head. Others were manacled to each other. Over the entry was the bust of the fat-faced, fat-lipped Pol Pot, the inscription scrawled over with a great cross. At the gateway was an inscription 'peace on earth.'

I never went to the killing fields of Choeung Ek, where those who were held in Tuol Sleng were killed. The total of those who died during Pol Pot's reign between 1975 and 1979 will never be known; but the Cambodian Genocide Program at Yale University estimates 1.7 million people, or one fifth of the population, lost their lives.

Pol Pot's regime had ended just twenty years earlier. Many people I worked with told me stories from that time. They were adolescents or older children with the resilience and strength to survive, but most had lost their families.

Later that day we had a meeting with the Australian High Commissioner in the embassy. It was a sanctuary, with high white ceilings, tasteful paintings, and expensive rugs behind huge block walls.

Besides Australia donors included Japan, France and the US with the US giving aid through nongovernment organisations (NGOs). There were 400 NGOs, mostly based in Phnom Penh, some of them shopfronts. Corruption was endemic and donors often built their own projects. Challenges included widescale logging, HIV/AIDS, and overfishing. Australia had a high standing as they didn't pull out during the political instability of 1997. The Commissioner warned us about violence and said there was no room for conflict resolution. If we were involved in, or witnessed a traffic accident, we were to get out. In rural areas people had been lynched.

Afterwards I went with another volunteer to Wat Phnom. People went to pray for good luck. I stood in silence before the altar, before a great glittering wild Buddha. We lit incense and I cried. I cried for the AIDS victims and myself, and for the break-up of my family. I was missing my sons. I looked downcast when I returned and one of the other volunteers asked why I'd come. I was getting too sluggish I said, and the world was calling me again.

That night I couldn't sleep, worrying about the appointment I had with Dr Tia Phalla, the Secretary of the National AIDS Authority.

The next day I found his office and knocked. As I entered, he looked at me. How unprepossessing I must have looked. A middle-aged, short, plump European woman with closely cropped black hair, travel trousers and a long-sleeved checked cotton shirt. Yesterday had thrown me and I was overwhelmed.

I sat down in front of him at the small desk. It was an unassuming office, but I had no time to survey it. The small intense black haired Khmer man in front of me took all my attention. He was also sizing me up. He settled back a little, and instinctively I felt I'd passed.

"I want you in Poipet," he said.

I'd read about that place in my 1996 Lonely Planet. The armpit of Cambodia they called it, the border town with Thailand, full of beggars, street kids, and corrupt officials, over 400 km to the Northwest. I sighed, hoping it didn't show. He showed me a black and white photo, a desperate woman pushing a huge cart.

"There are ten thousand border crossings daily," he said.

They were there because of the high tax on trucks.

"They think its heaven," he said, "But it's hell on earth, and they keep coming."

The health centre built for 5000, now had to cope with 40,000. MSF (Medecins sans Frontieres) was there, as was ZOA, a Dutch organisation.

I muttered something about Battambang.

"Battambang is stable," he said forcefully. "You are not needed in Battambang."

I looked at him, surprised at his confidence in me. Well, he has faith in me, I wish I had more myself, I thought.

Then he said, "Keep your eyes open and your mouth shut. You need a great heart."

I nodded. The interview was over.

Nothing could have prepared me for the reality of that place. It was as he described, and worse. But he had said enough. What had I got myself into? I went to Wat Phnom and circled it as I knew the locals did, hoping it was the right direction and praying. "God, Buddha, this is too big. We need your help."

That was a practice I continued. I sought solace in the temples, in my garden, walking in the rice-fields and walking in the hills. And yet he had faith in me, like my father, who when I'd vented had said, "You'll find a way."

As I left the temple, I saw a woman and her two children,

exhausted, sleeping beneath its roof. These were the people I was here for. It was not about me.

Friday at last, and I was relieved. That afternoon I boarded a plane. It landed at Siem Reap and I got off but was hustled back on by the hostess. The second and last stop was Battambang where a land cruiser waited. After driving through parched rice-fields we arrived in Sisophon in the late afternoon. At the CARERE (Cambodia Area Rehabilitation and Regeneration) Office I met the Director in the dark wooden reception area and followed him up the circular stairs.

The sun was setting as I looked out the window at the barren hill, a fort on top, with a flag flying. For two years I would be there. I felt I'd arrived at the ends of the earth.

The Director looked at me and said kindly, "It's alright. Most people feel like this when they arrive."

Chapter Two

POIPET, THE EPICENTRE

I was one of 10 expatriates living in a town of around 60,000 people. But where were they all? My initial impression was of a small town, perhaps 10,000 people. It was on the rice plains, with a river south of the town and hills behind. It had mostly dirt roads, peppered with ruts and potholes, which became impassable in the wet.

The Lonely Planet 2000 described it as a necessary, but uninteresting town, a service centre for Banteay Meanchey province, and a transport hub. Highway 5 led to Battambang 70 km away, and Phnom Penh, while Highway 6 led to Siem Reap. Both roads were awful, and it took over 22 years and $143 million dollars before the road between Sisophon and Battambang was upgraded. There was a provincial service centre, a market, a few temples, shops, hotels, restaurants, pharmacies, a health centre, an MSF sexual disease clinic, a military base, and brothels.

Sisophon was still unstable four years before I arrived. The Khmer Rouge and Cambodian troops battled for ascendancy with both sides committing human rights abuses. An official told me in 1996 he and his guests had to take refuge under a table when shooting started. But after the initial shock I grew to appreciate Sisophon. It was just 50 km from Poipet and the Thai border, and off the tourist track.

The Director orientated me physically and mentally, and I stayed with him and his family until I found my own house. He also provided fascinating insights into SEILA (Khmer for foundation) a program administered by CARERE. CARERE, funded by the United Nations Development Program (UNDP), supported the creation of elected village, commune, and provincial committees, with two of the five positions in village committees allocated to women. Besides good governance, the goal was poverty alleviation. It was also a framework for former Khmer Rouge areas as they became part of the country. The 1999 budget of US$2.4 million for Banteay Meanchey for three years funded farmer training, rural loans, health centres, schools, wells and latrines, literacy programs, roads, irrigation canals and demining activities.

These CARERE village and commune committees were the key to community mobilisation for the HIV/AIDS program. The leaders and members of these committees knew their village members and worked with us. This was critical in a country where the health services were often inaccessible or poor quality, and poverty and illiteracy widespread.

I arrived at the Director's house in the early evening and with his family sat down to homemade tomato soup and homemade bread. It was the first of many fine meals in Cambodia, some the best I've ever eaten. The French and Asian influence combined with the use of fresh produce, pounded with fresh herbs and spices, created a subtle, unique flavour. After the meal, exhausted,

I excused myself and went to bed with the direction I was not to use tap water to brush my teeth.

I instantly fell asleep in the comfortable bed next to an open window and woke in the early dawn. There was shrill nasal Chinese singing on one side, and on the other, clucking chickens. I became accustomed to weddings beginning at 4.30am next door, but the first was a shock. I soothed myself by eating my last muesli biscuit and reminding myself that just a week ago, I had flown out of Australia.

During that first weekend I stuck closely to the house, despite the Director's simple map of the town and the safety instructions accompanying it. Instead, I looked through the books and tried not to think too much about the coming week.

Monday came and I sat beside the Director in his land cruiser enjoying the high vantage point, looking down on a pony hauling a cart carrying a mattress. The horse trotted along, plumes on its head, bells jangling, while the lean driver leaned back bored, balancing on the narrow edge of the cart, his whip in hand. Women in long skirts and heels carrying laden nylon-net bags, picked their way along the dried mud footpaths. Motorbikes wove around the vehicles, men in caps and girls riding side-saddle in dark long skirts. Little ragged boys with huge sacks on their backs wandered along, poking at rubbish, and rifling through bins.

A policeman gave us a friendly wave and pulled over a laden ute. From behind came a siren blast, as a truck, its tray laden with a row of armed soldiers sitting stiffly back-to-back, pulled out of a side street. This was the Governor's army. An ambulance passed us laden with cheerful people. Unlike the truck with soldiers there was no siren, and they were probably going on a picnic.

On arrival I waited downstairs and found Poipet on the large map in the lobby dotted with flags. I was called upstairs and introduced to the health officer, a nurse. He was a shrewd, bespectacled man with a mop of thick black hair. After a tour of blurred faces and unpronounceable names we went to his office. He handed me some files and, while I studied them, tackled a cluttered desk and answered the constantly ringing phone. I learnt the Provincial AIDS Office had run the same low budget program for five years and it consisted of selected ministries giving a few talks. At least they had a good surveillance system supported by the CDC, or Centre for Disease Control and Prevention, but they had yet to tackle the data that emerged.

"Wow." I said wiping my brow. Sensing a presence, I looked up. There was the tea lady bowing meekly before me. Gratefully I accepted a cup of tea sweetened with condensed milk.

Fortified, I was driven to the Banteay Meanchey Provincial Health Department. As we passed a dusty pharmacy display featuring syringes, I looked at them nervously. In these countries they were often reused and became yet another source of infection. We stopped before a two storied building, with roller doors below and offices on top. We walked up the stairs and I met the WHO doctor. He had a larger office than Dr Tia Phalla's, comfortably furnished with a lounge and coffee table. I imagined a stream of consultants passing through however I was not one of them. I turned towards the European man, about the same height as me, also with dark hair. Unlike the consultants I was staying, and he looked at me critically.

"We expected you two days ago," he said.

"Sorry," I said. It was my habitual response although my arrival time was not something I could control.

He asked about my background in HIV and AIDS, and I said I had none. Quite reasonably he asked me what I thought I would do. I said I didn't know, but first I would meet the locals, and with them assess the situation.

"It's getting worse."

I nodded and said, "Yes, I spoke with Dr Tia Phalla."

That impressed him and he said, "The Thais are anxious. They don't want their people infected from this side of the border."

I asked him what was happening.

"One of the two effective NGOs is leaving the province and the other works independently of the Ministry."

"Right, and I see the PAS (Provincial AIDS Secretariate) program hasn't had much impact."

That was the name for the program featuring ministries and their annual talks. He nodded and invited me to attend cross border talks with the Thais the following week. I thought that was premature and told him my passport was still being processed in Phnom Penh.

"That's alright. We'll get you through."

Bluntly I told him I needed time to assess the situation.

I was then taken to meet the Director and Deputy Director of the Provincial Health Department. We entered an airy pleasant room with air conditioning and computers. The Director looked at me with polite anxiety while behind, a younger, smooth-shaven man burst into Khmer. The WHO doctor's interpreter looked uncomfortable when I looked at him questioningly.

"He says they have a lot of experience with AIDS and wonders why you've come."

"I was told this province has the highest positive HIV rate in Asia and it's increasing. Is that correct?"

The younger man spoke, and the interpreter said, "This epidemic has come from Thailand, and they're working with the Thais now. What will you do?"

"I don't know yet, but I'll work with my Khmer counterparts."

"Do you need an office?" the Director asked gently.

I nodded and followed him down the corridor. He unlocked the door and we walked into a small room with cracked and peeling plaster walls and one small high window. In the corner stood a broken chair. The light didn't work.

"That's alright," I said hastily, 'I'll sit beside the Director of the Provincial AIDS Office." I'd been told I would be his counterpart.

I left, followed downstairs by a tall, thin man with a large bunch of keys. He unlocked and rolled up the door, and I looked into a long dark room. Rays of sunlight, laden with dust, reached half-way, illuminating a large wooden table surrounded by old chairs. Nearby was a desk and on it, the oldest working typewriter I'd ever seen. Beside it were two large cardboard boxes with a stain emerging from the bottom of one. As my eyes adjusted, I saw fading photographs on the back wall labelled World AIDS Day. Cheerful Cambodians in AIDS Day tee-shirts held balloons. Above them, smiling benignly, were the Cambodian King and Queen, while on a large poster to the side a couple embraced. Below the man's muscled back, a condom packet peeked out of his jeans with the advice, 'Love carefully.'

I didn't hear him come in, but when I looked up, saw a small man with a youthful face. We shook hands and introduced ourselves. This was Eap, my counterpart. He bowed slightly and walked towards the typewriter.

Sitting down he asked, "Do you speak Khmer?"

"No, but I'm learning."

"Well, I don't speak good English."

"What's happening with that box of condoms?" I asked pointing to the stain beneath one of them. It was leaking, not a good sign.

He didn't reply. Instead, he began typing and said, "Come back when our workshop starts in a week."

Initially I was deflated but I recognise now it was the best thing that could have happened. I had to make my own way.

———

I was surprised when the CARERE Director asked me to go round the soldiers with an army nurse, but on Wednesday morning I drove cautiously to a military base on a motor bike I'd been loaned. I'd had lessons in Australia and practiced on gravel roads, but these roads with their potholes and unpredictable drivers were challenging.

I joined the man waiting for me and immediately felt at ease with his honest square face. Pulling the bike onto its stand, I asked why women were waiting near a small shed. He told me they were widows collecting their pensions. I asked innocently if their husbands had died fighting.

"No," he said shaking his head, explaining it was malaria, or AIDS. AIDS couldn't be mentioned though because they would lose the pension. I asked if many had died.

"Yes. That's why the General started a campaign with his own money and that's why you're here," he said.

I followed him on my motorbike, and as he sped off, I stopped and waited. He came back and I told him it was my first ride in Cambodia, so he slowed down. Those back streets with their wooden houses interspersed with shacks and a few dusty bushes, were where some of the sixty thousand Khmers lived.

He pulled up at a partly built house. The bottom floor had walls, but the top, just a floor and a roof. I thought it was deserted until a black-haired woman stood up on the far side and hurried towards us. Her hair was jet black and contrasted with her pale, deeply furrowed face. With a soft greeting she led us to a solitary bed.

The man propped up on the pillows looked like a cadaverous puppet. Even in the gloom his face looked blue, with the slow rising and falling of his chest the only sign of life. Beside him was a wooden dresser. The nurse and the patient's wife looked at me expectantly. I wondered what they thought I could do. He was dying. I took his hand and felt his pulse. He had a pulse, but his hand was cold, and his eyes closed. I wondered aloud if we could rouse him.

Even in Khmer I recognised the ritual squeeze, the command to name himself, but he remained unresponsive. Meanwhile I looked at the bedside photo, the well fleshed, proud military man, with a row of medals on his chest. His lank hair lay on the pillow and the nurse looked at me.

"We should put him on his side. He's unconscious," I said.

"I've told her before," he muttered, as his wife sailed in a with a cup of dark ginger smelling liquid on a tray.

"What's that?" I asked alarmed.

"Medicine."

"She's not going to give it to him?" I asked disbelievingly. "Tell her she can't."

The woman set the tray down and spoke sharply to the nurse.

"She's asking what we're doing," he said.

"He's unconscious for heaven's sake. She can't give him anything," I replied.

The woman watched her arms folded.

"She will," he said.

"I have to go," I said and stumped out. I couldn't watch that woman pour fluids down her unconscious husband's throat. I told him this when he reached me at the bottom of the stairs.

"Why did you bring me?" I asked plaintively.

"I thought you'd talk with her," he said.

"I would have if I thought she'd listen." As I got onto my motorbike, I thought, perhaps she's doing him a kindness.

The second patient looked at me suspiciously as I sat next to him on a wooden bench on his small veranda. He was wearing a faded tee-shirt and shorts and endlessly swinging his legs. I moved over when the nurse arrived. He greeted the man and almost apologetically handed him a packet of pills including vitamins.

"What about Bactrim?" I asked.

"You recommend it? For how long?" the man asked looking at me more amicably.

"For the rest of your life. It gives you protection, especially from a very bad pneumonia, as.."

I stopped and both men looked down,

"It, it's an antibiotic," I said stammering. "Quite cheap."

"Cheaper than those antiretrovirals?" the man asked bitterly.

He'd been an officer, and in the process of buying his two sons' lucrative customs jobs at the border, when he fell sick. Now his money had gone on cures that hadn't worked, including antiretrovirals from Phnom Penh. The supply had been erratic, and he couldn't afford to continue.

He fell silent and looked at the ground as he continued swinging his legs. Finally, he spoke again.

"He wonders who you are," the nurse said. "He thought you were from MSF."

"No," I said introducing myself.

The man looked at me disbelievingly "What do you do?" he asked.

"I'm still working on that. What do you want me to do?"

"Get me into a MSF program," he said earnestly.

"Did you ask them?"

He didn't reply. After we'd left the nurse explained. He'd approached MSF and been turned down. MSF did provide antiretrovirals in Phnom Penh at Preah Norodom Sihanouk Hospital, but not until July 2001. In 2000 antiretrovirals were still very expensive, US $10,000 per patient per year. People paid privately and the treatment was delivered in hospitals under medical supervision. Nowadays, with generic and mass-produced production antiretrovirals cost $63 per person per year.

I realise now how naïve I was. Instead of seeing the dying I should have asked to meet the General to discuss working with the living. Still there must have been some positive feedback to the Ministry of Defence because on my first visit to Phnom Penh I was invited to meet an official.

———

Finally, in the early afternoon on Thursday I arrived in Poipet with the health officer from CARERE. Never had I seen such disparity; beggars without limbs, skinny Khmers pushing carts, street kids and tiny girls with babies begging, while plump, contented Thais walked to the big new casinos.

This shantytown grew very quickly. A New Zealand volunteer couple who worked in Poipet in 1998 said the road to Thailand was then lined with shanties. There were no concrete buildings and when ZOA, the Dutch refugee support organisation arrived, they set up in a tin shack. It was the second grandest building in Poipet.

When the international border officially opened in February 1998, after fighting between the Cambodian army and Khmer Rouge had stopped, it was clear money could be made. The Poipet Military Police Commander built the first 49-bedroom hotel, the Neak Meas, for $400,000. There were plans for a casino and twenty thousand people arrived. It was clear even then land along the main road was valuable, and shanty dwellers were moved on. When I arrived two years later, Poipet's population had doubled to 40,000. The casinos were a great success as they were not permitted in Thailand. While I was there, there were six.

I wrote to the family after the first three visits that day. We were resting at the hotel to recuperate before going out at night, when Poipet really came alive. It was raining, but at least the rain would settle the dust churned up by the long convoys of trucks. The dust was so thick when we arrived the driver couldn't see.

Outside in the rain were thousands of people, and hundreds of children, with no shelter. Some lived under a bit of thatch, a piece of plastic or in a tiny leaf hut. The mud tracks through the interior of the town were much more treacherous than the four-wheel drive tracks in Australia. There were one or two drinking wells, no toilets and there had been a big cholera outbreak. On the main road were big new tiled buildings, the casinos, hotels, and massage and karaoke parlours, with fleets of trucks parked outside them.

Our first visit was to the MSF sexual health clinic. That was appropriate because since their arrival in 1998 they had reduced the sex worker's HIV positive rate from over fifty percent to thirty percent and condom use had increased. There were 20 brothels and 120 sex workers. It was a brutal trade with sixty percent of the sex workers either forced or sold to brothels. They were then bonded financially and unable to escape, even while they accessed MSF services.

The clinic was a high roofed, shed-like building near the market, partitioned and with an upstairs section. It was busy. They had up to five hundred visits from sex workers a month and visited brothels. The government clinic had about thirty visits per month. MSF also provided services to around 50 women who worked as beer and karaoke girls, and sometimes sold sex to supplement their incomes. These women were known as indirect sex workers or entertainment workers and were more difficult to find.

Sex was cheap, from $US0.5 to US$1, and the average number of clients per night for brothel-based sex workers was four. Many of the customers were labourers and cargo haulers, away from their families. The Khmer women, many of whom were illiterate and innumerate, made less than the Vietnamese, who were preferred because of their whiter skin and education. The Vietnamese were aware of what they earned and managed to save, unlike most the of the Khmers who remained in permanent debt to the brothel manager.

On National Women's Day MSF staff in Poipet invited sex workers to their centre, gave them a flower each and had vocational trainers available. A sex worker in her early thirties with three children wanted to give up sex work. Emergency housing was found, and her children were sent to Goutte D'eau, while she began vocational training.

We then visited Goutte D'eau, now known as Damnok Toek, where her children had gone. By the gate was a lovely child's drawing of the sun. The twenty-four children, some of whom were twelve to fourteen, made the thatch huts they slept in. They cooked for themselves, had a meeting hut, a dam for water and an open classroom. After six months they were sent to a vocational centre.

There were three four-year-old girls who'd been sent back from Thailand. One came up, and I couldn't restrain myself. I picked her up and carried her. She had a totally expressionless face, and I couldn't imagine the depth of trauma that caused it. When I set her down, I wondered if I'd done the right thing because I was yet another adult abandoning her.

There were more children at the drop-in centre supported by United Nations International Children's Emergency Fund (UNICEF). Outreach workers took food out to the street children. Sometimes they'd been recruited by a Fagin-like older child to steal, and they were encouraged to become glue sniffers. Sometimes parents needed or wanted their children to beg. Those rescued were sent to Goutte D'eau if there were vacancies, and sometimes sent back to their families.

I saw the harrowing nature of this work etched in the face of the expatriate UNICEF worker. She was exhausted. She gave grapes to a boy with no hands and a sick boy lying on the floor. She couldn't take him to the government clinic because it was rarely open, and they couldn't afford a private clinic. They took him to a private pharmacy hoping the drugs they bought were not fake.

This was my first experience of the major problem affecting government clinics and most government services, including police and teachers. Government workers were paid from US$8 to US$20 per month and had to resort to private work. It encouraged corruption and poor service provision in the government services; while to make a living Khmers ran private businesses, took bribes, tutored, or undertook daily work with Non-government Organisations or NGOs.

The hotel where we were based, had the narrowest corridors I've ever seen and was designed for sex. My small room was almost fully taken up by a queen size bed topped with a very hard mattress covered in plastic. There was a thin sheet, a towel-like blanket, and a red light. I lay down to rest when there was a hasty knock at the door. I got up and found my feet in two inches of water. The man next door had left his shower on. They mopped it up and I locked the door.

We had a meal in a nearby restaurant and went to pick up a worker from a local NGO. He was living on a plot of land with twenty of the poorest families. They each had a small house although the land was disputed. We walked around enormous potholes, full of mud. Gangs of sixteen-to-eighteen-year-old boys passed us while small children sat around a fire, sniffing. People lived in shacks and thatched houses with no light except what spilled in. Passing a shack the curtain briefly blew aside, and inside I glimpsed a wooden platform and a mosquito net.

We then went to see the Cambodian Women's Crisis Centre (CWCC) funded by Oxfam Hong Kong. It was founded in 1997 after the government temporarily closed brothels, then reopened them. The government was urged to do so by Dr Tia Phalla. He wanted sex workers to be recognised, so services could be provided.

There were four staff, a computer and three large folders named rape, trafficking, and domestic violence. They'd had a few rape cases in the past seven months but were constrained because only the government clinic could examine a rape victim and they were rarely open. One of their workers had been a police prosecutor and they had taken some cases to court. They'd had seventy complaints about trafficking in seven months, largely referred by suspicious neighbours, and had got the victims to safety. There was little chance of success with the court cases though because the traffickers were well connected.

After driving to the brothels, we found the girls sitting outside. As we walked through the streets, they hurled themselves at the men grabbing at their genitals. The health officer was targeted because he was chubby, wore spectacles and looked wealthy. We spoke with the girls, many of whom seemed drugged. The health officer said later that if they didn't have sex with four to five clients a night the brothel owners would beat them.

We passed a karaoke parlour with wide eyed boys and men watching sex videos in the sex café. The risk of these sex cafes only became apparent to me twenty years later after reading a warning by Ma Sameat of the Cambodian's Women's Crisis Centre. After the Ministry of Health HIV/AIDS testing centre and hospital was opened in Poipet in May 2003, it was found that in the previous two months between one quarter and one half of those tested were HIV positive and many did not have symptoms. Ma Sameat said this further AIDS awareness campaign, combined with the pornography and violence of the sex cafes, led to an increase of rapes with 14-to-15-year-old boys raping 10-year-old girls. She wanted the sex cafes closed and said she had lobbied the provincial and district heads. Both the Provincial and District Governors denied this.

While we were out a small woman came up carrying a mobile phone. She was from the Cambodian Human Rights and Development Association (ADHOC) and walked the streets at night finding domestic violence victims. There was a lot of violence associated with a drug called yama, a methamphetamine. We admired her courage and she said the police supported her.

On Saturday I woke up terrified. It wasn't a dream but the sense of an evil presence, something my Solomon Island and Maori friends would have understood. When I woke fully, I realised it hadn't harmed me and didn't mean to. It was curious. Still, I needed to recover and went for a walk.

Following a road up a hill I found a large truck blocking part of it. A woman crouched under it, collecting water in a bowl from the truck's underbelly and I hoped there was not too much diesel in the water. During the dry almost one third of rural woman in Cambodia collected water from rivers and streams, lakes, and ponds. This became increasingly difficult as these sources dried up or became more polluted.

At the top of the first hill was a monastery with orange robes hanging from the windows. I kept climbing, finally at peace in the silence of the hills and then heard hammering. I passed a shack, beside it a woman squatting, breaking rocks with a hammer, a couple of children playing in the dirt alongside her.

Further along I stood on a bluff overlooking the town, and followed the spine of the hill, towards the fort and flag I'd seen a week ago. It was a steep climb through the brown parched grass, but it was good. Metaphorically I'd been climbing all week and now I was climbing physically. At the top I looked over the burnt brown plains on the other side. There were fewer houses, the curve of a river lined by trees, and the roads with beetle-like vehicles.

Then I saw a statue behind me, a pilgrim brown and bearded, with a bare torso, a cloth around his waist and a staff in one hand. Around his other shoulder, hung a bag with a book. I looked at his wise and compassionate face, at his book bag, and contented stood alongside him, looking over the plains below. I'd found the solace I was seeking.

"I'll think of you up here, in the sun, in the wind, and in the storms, when life below seems overwhelming."

———

That evening, I went to a party marking the exit of HealthNet International (HNI) from the province, the NGO moving to the Vietnamese border the WHO doctor had spoken of.

I was sitting alone at one of the back tables away from the music and general jollity and thinking of leaving, when I noticed a woman nearby. A slender, attractive Khmer, dressed in an elegant silk skirt, she was watching her small daughter bouncing a balloon.

Impulsively I went over and introduced myself, asking if she was part of the organisation leaving. She said she was, she was Sarin, but she was not leaving. Her husband ran an orphanage in Sisophon and she would stay.

"What are you going to do?" I asked.

"Be a housewife."

"But aren't you a nurse?"

"A midwife."

"Do you know anything about AIDS?" I asked.

She nodded and said that in her experience there were two or three cases in each village. I looked at her and wondered if we could explore the situation together. I said nothing because I knew I would have to pay her. Did I have the money? How much would it cost?

The next day, Sunday, I woke up still thinking about her and I spoke with the Director. It would cost US$10 per day. I was determined to do it and did. Later the Brisbane Quakers supported the cost.

———

Meanwhile I'd begun walking around the town. There were buildings going up, even on Sundays. Bricks from the brick factory were taken to the building sites by pony carts. Labourers, many of them women in Vietnamese conical hats, built bamboo scaffolding, and hauled the bricks up in buckets. On top they slapped them together. Luckily Cambodia was not an earthquake zone. I also passed the ice factory which distributed large blocks of ice on the back of pony carts. Few people had refrigerators.

In the dry rice plains, there was still a small lake, a magnet for the people and wildlife around it. Vegetables grew on its banks and people waded in and cut lotus flowers. A small boy standing at the back of a narrow skiff punted himself with a pole, while others cast nets. Small boys herded oxen along the road. As I passed a group of huts people called out and asked why I wasn't on a motorbike.

My Khmer was good enough to hear their question, but not to reply that I loved walking.

———

In the middle of the next week, I had my first experience of the value of the SEILA structure. I visited a commune with the health officer, and we spoke with the commune chief. He told us there were around 1200 families in nine villages. Three of the villages had landless people with children who didn't go to school. Five people had died in the past year from AIDS and five had died from other causes. The five men who died had all worked as labourers in Thailand and their wives were sick.

A survey of 15,000 Khmer women in 2000 showed that 30% of women in Banteay Meanchey farmed their own land and 13% farmed family land. The rest had no land. During Pol Pot's regime land deeds were destroyed and those with knowledge of boundaries killed. When Khmers returned from border camps in Thailand there was a struggle to regain land, but much of it was heavily mined. Senior political and military personnel took possession of the more valuable land, and many families were left landless. To survive, members of these families were forced to migrate to Thailand for work. Away from their families, with cheap sex plentiful, the men were at risk of HIV.

The chief went on to say that in every village there were two to five people with symptoms of AIDS. Villagers avoided them because they didn't understand how HIV was spread. The chief thought the nurse should visit each village during the evening when people were home. Men and women needed separate awareness sessions, together with condom demonstrations. We spoke with the nurse, who said he needed training and more money. He thought villagers would buy condoms for 2 baht a box.

The commune chief asked that two monks from Wat Norea

in Battambang stay with his monks and teach them how to look after AIDS patients and their families. I planned to visit Wat Norea with Sopheap, the CARERE Religious Affairs Officer that weekend.

Later that day I went with the health officer to another commune. He and his team raced off and I stayed with the driver at the vehicle.

He was smoking and as he ground the butt under his shoe he asked, "Why didn't you go with them?"

I shrugged. The sky was hazy, the heat intense and I was sweating. The only sound was the oxen picking at the rice straw.

"It's cooler down there," he said, looking at the river. That was true although the water was now just a trickle.

On the steps of one of the huts an old woman was searching for nits in a child's hair. They both had a brightly coloured piece of cloth around their waist, the mark of the poor.

"What are you doing here?" he asked suddenly, looking at me suspiciously.

As I explained he was convulsed with laughter, and I looked at him surprised. Another driver had told him about the health officer's walk through Poipet and how the sex workers had grabbed at him. He recovered his eyes still crinkled in his broad face.

"You should talk with them," he said.

Suddenly he called out to the old woman. She stood up reluctantly, tightened her cloth around her, found her stick and hobbled over, the child and a mangy dog following her. He spoke, the child ran off, and slowly they gathered a dozen women of all ages, some carrying babies and others with children clutching at their skirts. They circled me and looked at me impassively.

I looked at the driver, he nodded, I began, and he followed.

No, they hadn't heard of HIV or AIDS except for a younger woman who had come from Phnom Penh. She spoke haltingly of what she'd heard. The others listened silently and then a darker older woman spoke up indignantly.

"She's asking what they're supposed to do," the driver said.

The woman spoke again, gathering speed, volume, and passion.

"They don't have condoms here and even if they did, they couldn't use them. Their husbands would beat them."

They stood around me silently. I sensed their fear, their powerlessness.

"We'll have to speak with the men," I said lamely.

The health officer returned and said there was no time.

I realised these were the women in my dream.

Chapter Three

A PROVINCIAL EPIDEMIC

B attambang, with its crumbling mansions and massive trees was pleasant and people happier too I thought, as Sopheap, the CARERE Religious Affairs Officer, and I bounced over the cobblestones of an arched bridge. Below naked children played and upriver a woman washed. Opposite her a woman drew water. Teenagers in white blouses, black skirts or trousers laughed and flirted at the riverside stalls, their motorbikes pulled up beside them.

Battambang was the second largest city in Cambodia, a transport hub between Thailand 110 km, and Phnom Penh 300km. There were tourists and it was possible in the wet to take a boat to Siem Reap. Many of the hotels and restaurants were remnants from UNTAC's time in the early nineties. There were 2 banks, a post office and many more NGOs than in Sisophon. The population in 2000 was around 120,000 people, twice that of Sisophon.

UNTAC (the United Nations Transitional Authority) arrived in March 1992 to stabilise the country before the first democratic elections in 1993. It was a US2 billion-dollar project involving twenty thousand foreign soldiers and civilians, and it spawned a thriving sex industry. Sexually transmitted infections increased sixfold between September 1992 and January 1993, including HIV.

Sopheap and I, had come to visit the monks at Wat Norea, the first temple in Cambodia to care for orphans and AIDS patients. The Venerable Muny Vansaveth established Norea Peaceful Children, to care for children orphaned by the fighting. In 1997 he included children orphaned by AIDS. Not only did he care for orphans and AIDS victims he also visited other wats and trained monks. Cambodia was the first Buddhist country in the world to develop a national Buddhist response to HIV/AIDS.

As we drove up from Sisophon, Sopheap told me about the ordeal he had endured to check his HIV status. Before marriage the government insisted couples tested negative. He had tested at three private laboratories and each time was positive. Finally, a friend advised him to get tested at the government laboratory in Battambang. He was negative.

This was a major issue. Arlys, an American who had worked with Khmers for seven years, ran a home care program in Mongol Borei, near Battambang. She told me later about a young man who was about to be engaged. He received a positive HIV result, and the whole village knew of it. He considered suicide and had emergency counselling. We needed accredited HIV testing laboratories in Poipet, Sisophon, and Mongol Borei and I raised this with the national team.

In Battambang I stayed with a volunteer and the next morning was woken at six by tinkling bells and a haunting cry. I crept downstairs, nodded at the guard and made my way into the street where I found a small boy with a cardboard box on his back. A woman stopped him, gave him a note and he handed over two French loaves. These bread vendors were walking alarm clocks and Edith, another volunteer who joined me later, found them annoying.

———

In the growing light there were joggers and walkers, while bike and car lights broke the gloom. Across the arched cobbled bridge came a line of monks, boys in orange robes, led by a small, ragged boy carrying a begging bowl. I gave him money as he gently bowed, and noticing the European behind him, looked at him enquiringly. This was Bob, an American, who lived with the monks at Wat Norea. I introduced myself and explained that Sopheap and myself would be visiting that day.

Later we walked down the road to the temple, past old stone buildings with orange robes drying from the open windows. A tiny woman with a shaven head in white robes swept the drive with a twig broom. The Venerable Muny Vansaveth was out and while Sopheap went to look for him, I asked about Bob. I was ushered into a cool lofty room where I admired the Grecian like stone pillars. Sitting on a bright cushion on an inlaid stone seat I looked at the photos, Gandhi, Martin Luther King and a monk. Long sky-blue drapes hung before the entrances and Bob, pushing one aside, entered.

He was weathered, spare and fit, a little taller than me and dressed in a tee-shirt and shorts. I asked him about the monk.

This was Maha Ghosananda, who with Bob, founded the annual peace walks (Dhammayietra), in 1992 when Cambodia was still at war with the Khmer Rouge. Bob was Bob Maat, a Jesuit monk who arrived in 1979. He worked in the border camps as a health worker for a decade before becoming a rice farmer in 1988-89. It was then he founded the Coalition for Peace and Reconciliation and met Maha Ghosananda. He said he had come to help, not only physically but spiritually.

"A country has to heal from its centre. That's why I came."

Most of the monks were killed during Pol Pot's regime; temples were used for killing and torture and Buddhist texts destroyed. When Pol Pot's regime collapsed in 1979, only 3000 monks of 60,000 in Cambodia in 1976, were still alive.

I followed Bob into the courtyard. We watched as two young monks flew past, orange robes streaming behind them, dribbling a soccer ball from one to the other. A pack of small boys pursued them valiantly, rushing between the two, but were always too late. Laughing, the barefoot monks disappeared around a corner, with the boys following, but they came back when Bob called them. They ran towards us and pulled up, giggling and chattering, then forming a queue bowed, and ran to get their food.

Bob collected a bowl from the women serving rice and vegetable stew and beckoned me over to a tiny shack. When I arrived, he'd disappeared inside. From the door I could smell the fug of an unwashed body and stale urine. Entering, I bumped into feet. As my eyes adjusted, I saw his skeletal frame, his face, while his eyes stared at me unblinking.

"Help me, he wants some water," Bob said. He was kneeling.

Bob tried to pull him up, but he groaned. Bob thrust a cup at me, and I left to find water. When I returned Bob had left and there were just the glittering eyes. I tried to sit him up gently and he groaned again. He was so thin, so fragile. He sipped the water and when a little spilled from the corner of his mouth, I wiped it with his sheet. When he'd drunk, he lay back exhausted, still looking at me.

"Sorry," I whispered.

He gave no sign he'd understood but closed his eyes.

After I'd left, I asked Bob how old he was.

"Twenty," he said. "He's just one of hundreds, one of thousands, some of them dying in the rice fields because they've been driven out by their families."

"How can I help?" I asked.

He wanted education pamphlets for the annual walk, the Dhammayietra, which took place in April. Hundreds of monks and supporters would walk across Cambodia, praying for peace, blessing villagers and leaders and drawing attention to Cambodia's problems, that year AIDS. I said I'd ask the WHO doctor and the doctors in the Provincial Health Department for help.

———

On Sunday I was back in Sisophon and woke at four to the nasal high singing of a wedding. I escaped and in the rice plains, caught the sunrise the red orb slowly and majestically squeezing over the horizon. A monk was chanting. At the end that road ended and there was a crossroads, so I turned to the right. A dog barred its fangs and barked. I stopped, acutely aware of rabies. A small girl passed and beckoned me through. Gingerly I followed and two small girls in uniform fell in step beside me. Although it was Sunday, some schools must have been open.

I pointed back to the dog, named it in English and in what I thought was Khmer. They corrected my pronunciation. I tried with coconut, tree, and other things we passed. Each time they corrected me. My daily lessons with my language teacher were going slowly. I needed to stop learning the script and start concentrating on the language.

The next day I joined the two-day PAS (Provincial AIDS Secretariate) workshop run by Eap, the Director from the PAO (Provincial AIDS Office). With a dozen others I watched as he paced in front of us speaking in Khmer. Opposite me at the long table was a media man in a flak jacket. He stared behind me, meditating on the fading AIDs Day photos. The pretty woman from woman's affairs studied her fingernails while others lounged or read under the table. I sat next to the Red Cross representative who had greeted me earlier in English.

"What's he talking about?" I whispered.

"Last year's program,"

I'd read about the $200 the ministries used for a few education sessions in villages. There was no evaluation and no follow up. It was as ephemeral as the dust dancing in the sunlight.

"Will they repeat it?"

He nodded.

It was pointless I thought bitterly. I'd spoken with Eap earlier about the importance of training the police, the nurses, the teachers. In Africa these groups were dying, and it would be the same here if they didn't wake up.

I endured the next morning and the afternoon, when they worked on their plans, everyone except for the two who got no money. They were the representative for rural development (whose brother had died of AIDS), and the representative from the Cambodian Mine Action Centre (CMAC)who told me they had one to two deminers dying monthly from AIDS.

———

At lunch time I went upstairs to speak briefly with the WHO doctor and advise him of my meetings and visits last week. When I told him the leaky box of condoms had gone, he said they'd probably been sold, and I felt guilty. When I told him of Bob's request, he gave me a pamphlet to discuss with the Deputy Director of Health.

I knocked on the Deputy Director's door and he opened it. He was furious but at least he spoke English.

"Who are you? Why have you come?" he asked.

"I'm a volunteer, here to help. I hate seeing people dying of AIDS."

I said this sincerely thinking of the general and the twenty-year-old in the temple hut.

He looked at me steadily.

I'd told him of Bob's request for pamphlets for the march and he'd told me he didn't have any money. I handed him the pamphlet the WHO Doctor had just given me. He said it was no good and he had a better one.

"Whatever you think," I said humbly.

He looked at me again. "You'd better be careful," he warned.

I wondered if he was referring to the military.

"I just help whoever asks," I said.

He looked at me again and his tone changing asked if I'd ever seen Mongol Borei. I wasn't sure what Mongol Borei was, but I knew I hadn't seen it, so I said no. He asked me if I wanted to see it. Yes, I did.

"We'll go then," he said.

"Good," I said, happy I wouldn't need to return to the workshop that afternoon.

I got into his sleek, low, powerful red sports car. I'd never ridden in anything like this before. He drove fast and well, weaving his way around the potholes, while on the other side utes, their trays heavily laden with people and belongings, blasted past. Leaning back in the bucket seat I felt I was being swallowed up by the road.

Before Battambang he took a turnoff, and we rode through a surprisingly large town, Mongol Borei. Then he pulled up on a semicircular lawn, behind which curved a large white building. The sign said it was a hospital, but it was quiet and there were no other cars. We walked through the double doors and met the Director.

It was extraordinary. There were no staff. Skeletal men and women, small children with bloated bellies lay on wooden beds with no mattresses. Occasionally a family member was beside them, but mostly they were alone. Very occasionally there was a bag of intravenous fluids hanging beside them.

The two men stayed outside while I went into a great

cavernous barn of a place. These were the HIV and TB patients. The floorboards were rotten, and I had to tread carefully. There were no windows and as I grew used to the darkness, I could see the inert skeletal forms lying there, some coughing. It was the Crimea again, except there was no Florence Nightingale.

I emerged from the dying and the darkness. I didn't know what to say. I didn't know what to ask. The two men looked at me and I understood why I'd gone in alone. There was active TB in there. I didn't care. I had faced that in the Solomons.

Our last stop was an airy clinic, where I met some nurses. A man was lying on a stretcher, each breath a gargantuan struggle.

'Help me, help me," he gasped. '

"We're going to give him some antibiotics," the Deputy Director said, and he did.

This was the first time I saw Pneumocystis Pneumonia, also known as Pneumocystis Carinii (PCP), a pneumonia caused by a fungus. Before antiretroviral use and the use of Bactrim it killed 75% of people living with AIDS. They caught it when their immunity dropped. Co-trimoxazole or Bactrim was used to prevent it was the medication I had recommended to the General. It reduced the prevalence of Pneumocystis Pneumonia to around fifty percent.

Back at the office I spoke with the WHO doctor. I said there didn't seem many staff there.

"What do you expect for $20 a month? We're trying to arrange for the World Food Program to feed them."

I was silent, still stunned.

"Well, it's been supported in the past and as soon as the NGO leaves it reverts back to what you saw."

"Can't anyone help?"

"In Thailand the monks are involved. I've always thought we could try that here."

I told him about Wat Norea and described the hut and the inmate Bob had taken me to see. Then I said, "In the New Year I'll go to Thailand and check out the monks."

———·———

On Friday 7th of April, the rain had stopped, and Sarin and I took a CARERE car out to Svay Chek. She had agreed to work with me for a daily rate of $US10. Svay Chek was both a district and a town which bordered Thailand and had no official border crossings. Much of the border was heavily mined and unpopulated. First, we picked up a nurse from the local clinic and then two policemen.

It was the worst road I'd ever been on. The driver continuously swerved around the huge potholes and sometimes barrelled through them. I was in the back seat and was asked to wedge the water bottles in the boot behind me more securely. As I turned around to reach them the cruiser bounced, and I fell sharply on the edge of the seat. I felt and heard my ribs crack and rolled back into my seat between the two policemen. I wasn't going to move again. This wasn't about the water; this was about me.

Outside was a moonscape, rocky, with stricken dried bushes and no sign of life. Twenty years ago, it had been a great forest with tigers and elephants. The only remnants were the logs for sale, stacked beside the scattered huts.

"What do they eat?" I asked.

41

"Roots, wild animals and birds if they can find them," Sarin replied.

I watched mud splattered people groping in ponds for fish.

Then we drove through a surprisingly prosperous village with solid timber homes, chickens, pigs and suspicious people. We stopped briefly and were told tersely by the headman that they knew all about AIDS and had nurses supporting them.

"Surely this is smuggling," I said back in the car. Sarin was silent and I remembered the policemen on either side.

The driver slowed for a checkpoint but was waved through.

"What's that about?"

"They're looking for logs."

"Bit late, isn't it?"

The border village where Sarin suspected there were people with AIDS was neatly laid out. Rows of pleasant timber houses were set well back from the straight smooth roads. There were dozens of houses, and more planned when they had finished demining. There were yellow ribbons strung across sections of uncleared land, while men in overalls holding metal detectors with probes, carefully and slowly scanned the cleared areas.

This system was ineffective, slow, and dangerous as it detected all metal. Between 1992 and 1998, 200 million pieces of metal were detected, of which just 50,000 or 0.3% were landmines. The workers were at risk of treading on the mines or prodding them too deeply. Following a demining accident in 2022 an official released figures stating between 1997 and 2022 154 deminers had been injured and 31 died.

We pulled up outside the largest house and trooped over

to sit in the shade beneath it. Sarin in her long blue skirt and white blouse was first to greet the man who emerged from the crackling radio room. Extending his hand, he greeted us with easy assurance and called for his women and children.

He told Sarin he'd lived there ten years and the village had grown from two families to one hundred. He spoke vehemently when Sarin questioned him and claimed there was no one with AIDS in his village. Most people were day labourers in Thailand. He said they knew about AIDS and wore condoms during sex. Deflated we retreated to the market to look for food and Sarin called the deminers over. They giggled and said they too knew about AIDS and its prevention.

After the meal, the headman and his family drifted away, and a group of women came up. Amongst them was one very thin woman. The others pushed her forward and she spoke slowly with Sarin. Sarin listened gravely then turned to me.

'She says she can't eat. First her husband died and then their baby son."

"Can she open her mouth?" I asked.

She did and we saw the thick white plaque on her tongue. This was thrush, common in people with AIDS. The women clucked sympathetically and began talking amongst themselves.

"They want us to take her to the MSF hospital at Thma Puok.

"Is it on our way?"

There was a protracted group discussion, and the woman was sent to collect her belongings. We were to drop her at the clinic on the main road, and I would give her money for transport. The woman sat behind between the two policemen and I moved into the front beside Sarin. We stopped frequently to allow the woman to retch.

Meanwhile Sarin told me how she survived during Pol Pot's time. She was ten and ran away with forty children to live in the forest around here. They'd lived on roots and berries and slept at night in tree shelters to avoid the tigers. Even now she was an expert tree climber. Malaria and starvation had killed all but four of them. Sarin ended up in one of the border camps where she met her husband.

"He's a very ugly man," she said proudly. "You can only trust ugly men. The others play around."

She told me it was years before they married because they were both the eldest in the families. Both had lost both parents, and it was their responsibility to ensure their siblings were educated. When they got married it took years before they had a child. Because she was a midwife and continually splattered with blood, she would not consent to become pregnant until she had had three negative HIV tests.

It was almost dark when we got to the clinic. As Sarin searched for the head nurse, I took the woman into the ward. It was a big room with white peeling paint, lit by a kerosene lamp. There were ten wooden beds without mattresses, two of them occupied. I gave her money for transport and the woman unrolled her mat on the furthest one and lay down, her bag a pillow, and an old cloth over her. I saw the fear in the other women's faces, and called the driver in.

They said there was another woman like this a few days ago and they knew it was AIDS. They asked how you caught it. They asked if you could catch it sitting behind someone on a motorbike or by shaking hands?

As I answered their questions, I watched their faces. As simply as I could I explained the disease and how it was spread. Their fear drained away. Their colour came back. They were not infected, not condemned to die.

As we drove back Sarin and I discussed it. I wondered how many other people were so afraid and so uneducated. We had found in most villages of around 100 families with an average of four children each, two to five people had died of AIDS and two to five people had AIDS symptoms.

We needed a meeting of all those involved. We needed to find out who was doing what and then I needed to go to Phnom Penh.

Chapter Four

PLANNING AND NATIONAL
SUPPORT – APRIL, MAY 2000

F inally, it was raining, there was thunder, and it was cooler. Writing to a friend I explained I was under a mosquito net because there were cases of dengue fever. A complication, more common in expatriates and children, was haemorrhagic dengue fever which could be fatal as it sometimes caused internal bleeding and shock.

I'd invited at least 15 organisations and ministries including monks to a provincial meeting after Khmer New Year. We hoped to identify the current services, gaps, the ways we could work together, and the training and resources needed. Then I would go to Phnom Penh to discuss the meeting outcomes with the UNAIDS Director and the National HIV/AIDS team.

During the holiday I moved into my own house, and I went shopping beforehand with my housekeeper, a stout, middle aged, imperious woman. She was almost trodden on by a tall, muscular, tanned American helping his elegant Thai girlfriend into a large land cruiser and for a moment she looked wistful. She had never married.

She took me to a market stall, and we had a wonderful meal, amok, a delicate fresh fish flavoured with herbs, cooked in banana leaves. Then we found a pony cart and overloaded it with a mattress, buckets, pots, plates, cutlery, chairs, and other household paraphernalia. The driver began to protest but retreated when confronted with her sharp blast. He sat resigned on the side of the cart his whip in the back of his pants and off we went.

Stopping before the gate of the two-storey wooden, blue house on the street corner we met the owner and unpacked. It was the courtyard that sold this house to me. While the upper veranda looked over the street, the lower one opened onto a garden with bananas, palms, and a pond. We were shown the western style toilet and shower I had requested, and I asked about the electric point for the fridge coming from Battambang. My housekeeper asked for a food safe, and the owner agreed.

Sarin and I also had a test run on the motorbike I had been lent. After an hour of driving, trying to avoid the enormous ruts, I was shaking. On the way back there was a brief shower and we got stuck as the mud jammed between the tyre and the axle. We had to scrape it out to get moving again. Then the choke button and horn fell off. It was a little 100cc step through.

My former host, the CARERE Director spent 3 days up at the Laos border with the Khmer Rouge in Oddar Meanchey. It was a province created in 1999 when the fighting stopped. After a morning's work he'd found $50,000, 7 tonnes of rice and large numbers of rice seedlings. He was also facilitating negotiations. I was beginning to understand how the right leadership and right connections were powerful and could transform these people's lives.

———·———

I walked down to meet the 500 to 600 monks who'd gathered in Sisophon on Sunday the 9th of April. They had gathered from four different directions and looked so hot standing in the pitiless sun during the speeches. These were the monks we had printed the pamphlets for.

I was standing at the edge of the crowd when the organiser beckoned me over. He was sitting in the shade of a pagoda with the senior monks. I was asked to give a speech and decided to keep it brief. I welcomed them, explained who I was and said, "I pray like you, that peace will continue, that you will be strong, and your country will prosper. I join you too, in hoping that trees will no longer be cut, and replanting will begin. I hope we can work together to stop the spread of AIDS, and care for, and show compassion to, those people living with it and their families. Thank you."

———·———

Khmer New Year was almost upon us, the equivalent of our Christmas, and I wondered what I would be doing. I didn't want homesickness to overwhelm me again.

On Wednesday afternoon Sarin invited me to join her family and the orphans for a picnic at the wat the next day. The next morning, April 13th, I arrived at her terrace house. Parked outside was a large truck with a crankshaft and an exposed engine. The back was already loaded with people. I climbed up, we drove to her husband's orphanage and picked up ten children. I then moved into the cab to join the family. Sarin was breastfeeding her two-year-old daughter, and I caught her husband's glance.

The tenderness she had for her child, and the love her husband had for both, was very clear. It was a slow but enjoyable ride and we often stopped to replace the fan belt. It had rained, the rice fields were greener and beginning to flood. People were looking for frogs to eat.

We arrived and we walked up the hill to the wat. Next to me was a boy with a bad cleft palate, and a little girl about six. She watched Sarin and her family with great sadness. Seeking comfort, a small boy curled up in the arms of the elephant god overlooking the flooded rice plains. Amongst the many small temples and shrines were dwellings for nuns, older women in white robes with shaven heads. Unlike the monks they could not beg for food and relied on donations. I asked Sarin about the gold leaf boat in the temple. It was a boat that carried the souls of the dead across a river to the underworld, like the river Styx in Greek mythology.

We sat down to barbecued chicken and rice, and a tasty green pawpaw, cucumber, and ginger salad. Sarin had her fortune told. She picked a token from a book, touched it to her head and then handed it to be read. She was told she would have a very successful year.

When I got back in the afternoon I went for a walk. Hearing noise from a temple I went to investigate. It was just after 4.30.

The women at the gate told me to go in. There were men banging drums, playing traditional instruments, and dancing who beckoned me over. I was the only woman dancing with about 20 men, while the women and children watched. This was New Year proper, as midnight was for us. I enjoyed it and hoped I hadn't broken too many cultural conventions. I was grieved that people were trying very hard to speak with me, while I struggled to understand and reply.

It was a still a holiday, so the next day I climbed a hill that I hadn't explored before. On top I saw stone steps going down into a limestone cave and following them emerged into a grotto. The sky was on one side while on the other was a big limestone overhang and a statue of an elephant. Under the overhang was a bed with a mosquito net, its legs in tins of water. There were several monks chanting and the oldest threw holy water over me.

That evening there were fairy lights, like ours for Christmas. Like Christmas too I had lovely food, beautiful mangoes Sarin had given me and lychees.

I used that holiday to unpack and move into the lower floor. The upper floor I kept clear for Edith, another volunteer who joined me in late June. I cleaned the small altar, decided I would buy some incense and I put my pictures and photos up. These were part of me, and wherever I was, turned the house or the room into a home.

I decided on my breakfast, hot bread from the bread boy, fresh bananas, possibly a pineapple, tea, and milk if I could find it. On Sundays after a leisurely breakfast on the veranda, I would visit the cave temple and visit the orphans. The next day I took the orphans seeds; tomatoes, beans, and pumpkins; seeds I'd brought over from Australia. As if to congratulate me a small girl brought me flowers.

———

The next day, Tuesday we had the provincial meeting. Most of the 15 stakeholders I'd invited came. It was well attended but I was shocked at how little was happening. I drafted a report for Phnom Penh, and we agreed to keep meeting monthly. That group became the AIDS Technical Working Group.

Sarin and I were in Poipet on Friday 21st of April, following a request from Cambodian Family Development Services (CFDS). CFDS supported vulnerable families with emergency support, income generation and food security but found it challenging meeting the complex needs of families living with AIDS.

The first family was headed by a widow who looked healthy, but her husband had died of AIDS two months earlier. Their four-year-old child died before him. The two-year-old had thrush and a big suppurating abscess behind his ear, both symptoms of AIDS. The government clinic was shut, and there was little point sending them to the Mongol Borei district hospital as I had discovered. I knew there was a MSF hospital at Thma Puok and Sarin and I felt this would be the best option if the family could get there.

They lived in a tiny platform house, and as we were quite a large group, I worried it would collapse. Around us were similar houses sitting in a swamp of unhealthy-looking water. They paid 2 baht to go to the toilet and paid to draw water from the well.

The woman worked every day sewing in Thailand and left the child with a sallow looking one armed woman. She lost her arm when she was attacked years earlier.

A thirteen-year-old cared for her siblings in another family, as their mother was in hospital. One of her younger brothers had a deformed foot and was in the orphanage at Sisophon.

We then saw a recently widowed woman who had had been sick since giving birth and looked anaemic and bloated. She had pre-eclampsia during pregnancy. While Sarin and I discussed the possibility of TB, the others considered how much rice to leave. A fly was sitting on the teat of the baby's bottle, and somebody hastily covered it. At least the baby looked OK.

CFDS agreed to refer these cases to Tess from Family Health International (FHI). It was difficult for local NGOs providing general emergency support during an AIDS epidemic. FHI was an international NGO with expertise in HIV/AIDS and Tess was very capable. We had lunch with her, discussed the referrals and she was happy to take them.

Then we watched street kids sniffing glue and went to Goutte D'eau. We were told between 400 to 500 children disappeared every month from Poipet into the brothels of Bankok. An experienced social anthropologist and consultant Graham Forde told me the following year, it was difficult to determine the numbers of children and adults who were trafficked. There was strong legislation and heavy penalties, but because of the high profits and corruption, the legislation was not enforced.

We also spoke with the Director of ZOA, a Dutch NGO. They had settled 2000 families in Poipet, built small houses and given them plots. As the fighting finished and the land was demined, valuable land was often grabbed by politicians and soldiers and the villagers driven off. There was more demand as soldiers demobilised, and now another 3000 families needed houses and plots. ZOA also drilled for water and encouraged families to build latrines as they had already had cholera outbreaks. Latrines were most uncommon in rural Cambodia in 2000 and most families didn't have them.

On Saturday the day before I left for Phnom Penh, I found people had changed. Instead of calling me barang, or European, people wanted to know my name. As the fields flooded, they opened the gates and caught fish in the fish traps, tiny little silver ones. Town children came to surf the water as it surged through, while families did their washing. There was a festive air with balloons, and I shook many children's hands. I had missed the sea and here it was, an inland sea, reflecting the trees and the clouds. As I began walking back it began to rain and a motorbike stopped. The male driver offered to unload his wife and small child and carry me. I absolutely refused.

Sarin stopped the small girl from bringing me flowers. She didn't go to school, the owner of the house didn't know her, and she didn't live where she said she did.

I woke on Sunday morning, April 23rd with a vivid dream. I dreamed of Sue, my 41- year-old sister whose death had sparked my mid-life crisis and my dream of the Asian women. She looked alive and happy. It was Easter Sunday and in this Buddhist country I hadn't even realised it. It was such a joy, and I realised I was like my father. After Sue's funeral, and while we walked along the beach he said, 'She's not dead to me, and neither are the others.'

I flew to Phnom Penh and stayed with a hospitable and kindly volunteer couple. I borrowed their old bicycle but found it challenging riding in the chaotic traffic. Aside from my host, I never saw another European on a bicycle.

On Monday the UNAIDS Director Geoff Manthey greeted me with the word "Saviour".

I felt uncomfortable because I was simply following Dr Tia Phalla's instructions to keep my eyes open, my mouth shut, and attempting to identify the unmet needs. Still, they must have been relieved. They'd hoped by feeding me into the situation I'd unblock the barriers, and I had. But there was a lot of work to do as I said when I gave him the stakeholder meeting's assessment.

I was shocked at how little was happening. Apart from MSF, FHI and ZOA and other NGOs working in Poipet much of it was arbitrary. It was not covering the high-risk groups such as the military, or any other high-risk areas, besides Poipet. At that stage we didn't know where those high-risk areas were. Another priority was to learn about home care. The hospital system could not absorb the tsunami of AIDS patients, and our referral hospital Mongol Borei was awful, as I'd discovered.

On Tuesday I went to the Calmette Hospital where they had an inpatient and outpatient program. I met a French doctor who taught HIV positive women how to make quilts and dishcloths to earn a living. Most patients couldn't afford antiretrovirals.

Taking a break on Wednesday morning I went to the hairdresser and bought myself some second-hand books. I had been thinking about some of the NGO officers I'd met. Their lives were pleasant, but they were cut off from the rural areas where 84 percent of the population lived. It was a brief break, enough to realise how personally I was taking the epidemic. It was hard not to, witnessing that needless death. I watched the seagulls flying above the roofs and longed for the sea and silence.

I was advised not to go out on Friday the 28th, because a march was planned by the Vietnamese. It was feared there would be violence, but ironically, I had an appointment at the Ministry of Defence. It was a huge multi storied building and I was told defence had a large budget. Indeed in 2000 it was US$ 100 million. The first challenge was to get in as there were four soldiers with AK 47s. I parked the old bike behind them and explained I had an appointment. They looked at me suspiciously but checked and let me through.

It was Kafkaesque. I wandered past room after room and finally on the second floor found an officer waiting for me. I don't know now what we talked about. He must have been vetting me and it worked. When I returned, I found while Eap and I were allowed to follow up the military, although Sarin wasn't.

I liked Sopheap, the Religious Affairs Officer from CARERE. I felt we had a spiritual connection. This feeling deepened when I attended the farewell party for CARERE on Saturday 6th May. He sang with such longing and tenderness, and evoked the plains, the green flooded rice fields, and the rhythm of life. I asked him about the song, and he said he'd first sung it in a border camp overlooking Cambodia. Never again did he want to see his country go through what they had. CARERE didn't leave but localised and when the Australian Director went to Phnom Penh, the health officer took his role.

When I saw Eap again, he expressed concern about me and said I was to rest more. I was getting too many wrinkles around my eyes. Meanwhile Sarin had arrived in Phnom Penh for HIV/AIDS training and later I learnt her niece Sopheak was with her. She worked with me when Sarin found other work and was a determined and effective educator. Sarin remained a good friend and I was always grateful for her support.

On Tuesday 16th May I went out with the home care team based in the Moung Ruessei district of Battambang. It was a pilot program run between the Ministry of Health and the AIDS Care Unit of NCHADS. Ten of these home care programs were based in Phnom Penh with one at Siem Reap and another at Battambang. Each program had two government nurses working part time and 3 NGO staff.

In Battambang the NGO staff were from KRDA or the Khmer Rural Development Association. Staff carried simple medicines in home care kits, visited clients three times a month, provided palliative care, and support to their families. There was a monitoring committee. KRDA staff told me they had 81 patients and visited them weekly.

It was an impressive program, the nurses were organised, efficient and compassionate. However, the person I admired most was the young women with HIV who accompanied them. I got to the KRDA office early and she let me in as she lived there. As she told me her story through an interpreter she began to cry. Her husband died of AIDS and their four children aged between 4 and 10 were with her mother. She didn't want to see them again. I held her hands, looked into her eyes, and admired her courage. Every day she was with these patients she was reminded of her own fate.

The first patient lived in a tiny wooden hut amongst a few others in a dry riverbed. He'd been a soldier and returned to his mother when he got AIDS. There was another patient, a young girl lying in a big open shed next to a rice mill. As I watched her raising herself on her elbows to swallow a pill, I sensed the sadness of the young volunteer alongside me.

There was a woman with two teenage children at either end of her mat, a boy and girl. They looked at her so sadly, willing her not to die. Their father was already dead. We found a big packet of pills beside her, which the nurse said were steroids. The dose was large enough for horses.

One woman we saw had three children and couldn't lift her head up for more than 15 mins without vomiting. She'd spent all money on medicine including what looked like steroids. She didn't trust the pills anymore.

This problem of inappropriate treatment from both private pharmacies and Kru Khmer or traditional healers continued throughout my stay in Cambodia. Because public clinics were rarely open and people didn't know what they would be charged, less than 5% of patients went to them. Two thirds either went to a traditional healers or private clinics and both could be lethal.

Arlys, who ran a home-based care team in Mongol Borei, knew of one family who had paid a traditional healer $3000 for 2 months treatment. Other AIDS patients had died from diarrhoea and vomiting after taking traditional treatment. It was suggested health centres and NGOs seek traditional healers and possibly community elders to assist with separating the good practitioners from the harmful ones.

We continued all day. Most of the patients were women, their husbands already dead. The program had support from a good district hospital. All the patients received Bactrim to decrease their chance of getting PCP, but antiretrovirals were still too expensive. As we drove back a small girl called from an open doorway and glancing at the young mother beside me, I saw her wistfulness, her sadness.

The hopelessness and sadness of that time would be echoed in the COVID-19 pandemic before effective vaccines were developed. We tried to provide the best information and care possible for the dying and their families, and at the same time worked on saving the living. It was difficult for many to accept there were no miracle cures. Those who knew more about the disease and were supported by their family and friends, had a better chance of dying peacefully. My heart went out to that woman. She must have died many years ago.

These women had been infected by their husbands. In a survey of 15,000 women carried out in 2000 it was found that nationally, a third of women would not refuse sex with their husbands if they were HIV positive. In Banteay Meanchey, almost half, 47% would not refuse sex with their husband if he was HIV positive.

It showed how powerless these women were, particularly in the rural areas. Over half had witnessed AIDS deaths, and births and deaths of sickly children born to infected mothers.

The next day Wednesday while I was still in Battambang I met two volunteers for Buddhism for Development. This organisation was formed in 1990 by monks in one of the Thai border camps, and when they returned to Battambang in 1992 they based the NGO at Wat Anlongvil. They supported sustainable socio-economic development. The volunteers worked in several villages, supporting people with transport to clinics and the hospital. Income generation schemes, such as raising pigs and selling food were also supported. It was uplifting to find faith-based organisations supporting vulnerable villagers. The organisation began another branch in Oddar Meanchey in 2001 and Pailin in 2003.

—·—

It was finally confirmed by both the WHO doctor and the CARERE Director that Geoff Manthey the Director of UNAIDS was coming, and he arrived on the 31st of May. I was very glad to see him in Banteay Meanchey. I asked him about increasing the nurses' pay, and he said it was unsustainable. The only way forward was to mobilise communities.

On the 2nd June it was my birthday and we celebrated it in

Poipet. Geoff Manthey, the Deputy Director of Health, myself, and the team had a meal in a casino, and the Deputy Director paid. Things had really turned around. It was a celebration, not only of me but our solidarity.

Poipet was growing. The Holiday Palace began operating in 1999 and was followed by seven others in the next two years. They catered not only for the Thai's gambling addiction but the Cambodian government's desire for cash. Around 1000 Thais daily crossed the border to gamble, and in 2001 the Cambodian government collected around $US4 million from the casinos.

As we emerged from one of the casinos, I saw a young woman carrying a baby. There was such despair in her eyes. Poipet was a complex town and prevention was difficult. Men were away from their families, sex was cheap, and according to the UN in 2003 up to 75% of the labourers and construction workers took cheap yama, an amphetamine to sustain their long hours and income. Fuelled on yama they tended to tear the condoms off, or not use them at all. Street kids became addicted to sniffing and made money to buy inhalants by smuggling clothes from Thailand. They were fodder for traffickers. Meanwhile the hierarchy profited from both trafficking and the casinos.

But it was a time for a break. It was time to leave these intractable problems behind, at least for a week. I crossed the border.

Chapter Five

A HOLIDAY AND A WORKING HOSPITAL – JUNE 2000

O n Sunday the 4th of June, overnight in a tent in a national park in Thailand I listened to whoops and howls, perhaps monkeys? There was also a mini-circular-saw like sound which grew louder and softer, and all the while the rain drummed down. But the tent worked, like so many other things in Thailand.

I was suffering from culture shock. In Poipet, while vehicles had been up the tops of their tyres in mud, people pushed carts and street children begged, I watched men building a brick tower. Standing on rackety bamboo scaffolding, they threw the bricks up to the next level. In Sisophon, they were more safety conscious, and hauled them up in buckets. After running the gauntlet of the beggars and customs officers, I passed under the arch, across the bridge and into Thailand. On either side streams of people were entering illegally, in full view of the customs officers.

Suddenly I was on a tar sealed road and there were tuk-tuks, plump contented people, teenagers in school uniforms and just a few motorbikes. There were no pony carts and there was no rubbish. I got a lift in a BMW. I wouldn't have dared hitchhike in

Cambodia, but here I was told it was safe. When I was dropped off, I got another lift on a motorbike. The young man dropped me at the turnoff to the park, and a couple drove me to the campsite. Humans were not the problem, instead it was the tigers, and the elephants.

After breakfasting I got another lift to park headquarters, 8 km from the campsite and took the track to the wildlife observation tower. It was midday, the sky was dark, the jungle dense, and the track muddy. It began to rain. After a couple of hours, I turned back, still 2 kilometres away from the tower. In the torrential rain I thought of Sarin and wondered how she survived three years in the jungle, while I was struggling with one day.

The rain stopped and back on the road I saw my first wild gibbon. As I looked at his wise patient face, he flickered his brow and blinked his yellow rimmed eyes. Behind him I saw the troop, the young swinging on thin branches and leaping to safety when they broke. There was a mother with a small baby clinging to her. I felt something trickling down my right leg. It was streaming with blood. The leeches had got me. Behind me a car stopped. Four young girls came over and offered me a large pair of white cotton stockings. I refused these, but gratefully accepted the toilet paper and the lift back to my campsite.

The last morning of my stay was glorious. It was fine and I walked down to the river. Out of the bamboo thicket shot a curious animal, neither goat, sheep, nor pig but the size of these. It was square and a warm brown colour. I felt I had just stepped out of the pages of Dr Doolittle, the story of the vet who talked with animals and housed a large and extraordinary menagerie.

I packed up and walked down the road sadly. In Cambodia trees, birds, animals, and even insects, had such a short life span.

Passing through Poipet on Friday the 9th I passed a young man with a wooden yoke across his shoulders carrying a huge load. He took jerky controlled steps, his back and face soaked with sweat. As he dropped the load, I watched his face. Release!

The street kids were playing at the edge of the sprawling market, while a man with no legs quietly drew on a cigarette. Together we watched a small girl carrying a laden backpack made of rice bags. Cargo haulers they called them. In Thailand she would have been in school.

It was good to be home and on Sunday I walked through the rice plains to a village with a store, a few pigs, a school and a wat. I sat down and talked with a schoolteacher who'd taught there for 20 years. My Khmer was good enough to learn he was 52, there were 426 children in the school, and he was responsible for the library.

At last, my daily Khmer lessons with my language teacher were bearing fruit and I tried speaking with the guard as well. I'd lost my housekeeper as I couldn't afford both her and Sarin. As I shopped, I chatted in pidgin Khmer with the market vendors. They tried to teach me about cooking the various lentils, and how to assess and cook different types of rice. I asked them about the different herbs and the various greens. Later I learnt to be careful of the vegetables because some were sprayed with toxic pesticides by illiterate farmers. These pesticides were banned in European countries.

On the 14th of June I went with the Director of CARERE to look at a community forestry project and clinic. We took the new laterite road to Phnom Srok.

Two to three years earlier this country had been held by the Khmer Rouge. The road was empty, but in the rice plains women were transplanting seedlings. They stared at the car and we passed a village surrounded by goats. Goats are a great source of meat and milk and very hardy. I hadn't seen them elsewhere and wondered if people from former Khmer Rouge areas were more enterprising.

We arrived at the clinic. It was shut but a staff member living nearby saw our vehicle and came over. Six nurses were supposed to work there, but only three were listed. They didn't have the 30 essential medicines deemed by WHO in country as necessary in public clinics. It was unclear if they'd been stolen, been sold to private pharmacies, or had never been sent. Generally, the country list includes staples such as antibiotics, antimalarials, TB treatments, oral rehydration sachets, analgesics.

We passed a village where children were being immunised and I hoped a sterile needle was used for each child. A couple, two teachers who'd volunteered in Africa previously, told me at my orientation in Melbourne, that a whole class they'd taught had died of AIDS after a vaccination campaign.

We lost the road and drove through scrub which came over the bonnet. There were large igloo shaped termite mounds and girls with baskets gathering bamboo shoots. Finally, after finding the road again, we arrived at the village with the community forest. It consisted of a few scrawny trees which the villagers were guarding.

The next day, I was out in the villages with one of the male Provincial AIDS Secretariate representatives for village awareness sessions planned during Eap's workshop. By the afternoon he was beginning to relax and following Sarin's example with the women, talking with the men and answering their questions.

———·———

On Sunday the 18th June I wrote to John my younger son:

People are dying of AIDS in the villages. There are also problems with drug addiction, yama, an amphetamine, sexually transmitted diseases, TB, malaria, and dengue fever. The list goes on. Despite this there is hope. People work hard, and there are very clever and determined people working alongside me, and in charge. We are working on proposals including village education and home care, schools and youths, risky border areas and vulnerable women. Besides the sex workers, the wives of soldiers, police and deminers are at risk. There is widespread infidelity and sixty percent of the men use brothels.

I take it day by day and get on with everyone. I am trying to fade into the population and lose the patina of the expatriate. I do my own cooking, go to the market and persist with trying to learn the language. I try to speak with my guard. I have found one road I can run on in the morning, a laterite road. The rest are too muddy. It was lovely to see an unpicked flower by the roadside this morning. Usually they're picked and sold.

The food is very good, although you have to get used to the newly butchered meat lying on old wooden tables at the market, with a few flies around. I try to buy it early. I still haven't worked out how to cook the fish. They come from small ponds and taste very muddy. There are all sorts of odd vegetables and one day I saw a lady selling fried grasshoppers. All the water must be boiled, and Giardia is common. There are very few toilets so sometimes the wells get contaminated and there are cholera outbreaks.

The Provincial Staff have gone away for a week so I'm going up to Thma Puok tomorrow to develop some proposals as requested by the UNAIDS Director Geoff Manthey. While I'm away I'm lending my motorbike to the man responsible for HIV/ AIDS in the education department. He's going to investigate the situation in schools but needs $US 5 a day. Sarin will go with him and needs $US 10 a day. Luckily the Quakers have given me some money for two months.

I arrived in the grey of very early morning at Thma Puok on Monday, the next day. The cocks were crowing and there was a strange ruin near the governor's house of great stone crumbling blocks. At the hospital, a great wooden shed, I toured with the MSF doctor. The common problems were upper respiratory tract infections, gastrointestinal problems, TB, AIDS, dengue fever in children, and malaria. Many of the HALO deminers working in this area got malaria the previous year. This malaria, like the malaria in Pailin, a former Khmer Rouge area, was multidrug resistant. The doctor told me medical assistants trained in border camps were being replaced by young doctors with seven years of training, but sometimes little clinical experience.

The rows of iron beds ran the full length of the ward. It was gloomy with a strong smell of disinfectant. Women and children lay on red rubber mattresses with sometimes a scrap of grey sheet, while relatives with bed rolls and pots slept on the floor. I saw two nurses, one hurriedly stacking files for the doctor's round, while the other hovered over a baby with a high-pitched wail.

We began passing from one stricken form to another. In a small side room, a child with severe malaria was fighting for his life. Another nurse was with this child. In the chair sat his silent, exhausted mother. She looked barely sixteen. The rate of malaria was much higher then. In 2000 the incidence of malaria was almost 81 per 1000 in populations at risk. Many people died because of drug resistance, the lack of second line treatment, and fake drugs.

There was a woman with beriberi, or lack of vitamin B1, who was comatose on admission. The doctor said these cases were increasing and it was unfortunate they removed the full husk in the rice mills, as it was the husk that contained Vit BI.

The children were heartbreaking, newborns looking like little old men, and toddlers too weak to walk with nasogastric tubes, swollen bellies, and emaciated limbs. The doctor gently turned a child's head, exposing a large abscess. She said she had drained it, would drain it again and he was on antibiotics. She suspected he was HIV positive, but it was difficult to diagnose in children under two. Two women were dying of AIDS, one with a son under two who may have had AIDS. The cook's wife was looking after him.

The veranda was warmer with more windows and the sun streamed in. This was where they kept the infective cases, the TB. I thought back to Mongol Borei hospital, the gloom of that dark cavern, the inert forms, and the coughing, and understood why villagers preferred this hospital.

In a tiny dark room, a man was struggling to breath. His torso was covered with sweat and every muscle was straining. His face was tense, his breath coming in great gulps. He tore off his oxygen mask and begged, "Help me, help me." The nurse came in, helped him put his mask back on and adjusted his IV.

"AIDS, Pneumocystis Carinii," the doctor said outside.

I nodded and replied, "I know. I saw another patient at Mongol Borei."

At the end of that first day I was dropped, with my bag, at the end of a long gravel drive. On either side was an orchard with ancient trees and long grass. I heard the cackle of geese and saw their furrows. There were crickets and a few birds. At the end of the drive two dogs on leashes strained and barked frantically. As I drew closer, they were pulled inside. Along the sides of the orchard was a moat bordered by poplars, their shadows long in the late afternoon light. Around a bend was a small cottage and behind it a timber house. As I walked up to the house, I heard radio static and a European male voice repeating a call sign. I knocked on the open door and was handed a key to a room in the cottage. I slept well. How could I not in such a peaceful rural setting?

Later I learned it was more dangerous than it seemed. Although it was safe in the day it was not at night. A couple of NGO workers were shot by bandits a couple of weeks after my visit. They were on a motorbike at 7pm just out of the main town.

On Wednesday I accompanied a Thma Puok District AIDS Officer out to Boeung Trakoun, a border town. We left at 7am on his motorbike. As he drove through the scrubby landscape he spoke of the unreported malnutrition, and the disinterested nurses. It was hard when they were not paid a living wage.

We stopped in the villages. The women were very worried about the risk of catching AIDS from their husbands. One pregnant woman said she thought of little else. We talked about rehearsing condom negotiation. Back on the bike the officer said to me, "If a man really loves his family, he will consider protection."

A village leader asked us many questions about private pharmacies. I told him it depended on who owned and ran them. Sometimes it was nurses and sometimes it was people with no knowledge or experience. They all sold a wide selection of medication and equipment, some of which could be lethal, and some simply unnecessary. There were also many fake drugs, which looked real but did not contain the essential ingredients.

After we returned, I walked down a mud street. On either side were brown thatched houses with no fences. There were a few ox carts with huge wooden wheels, the driver riding on top with a whip. At the end of the road were giant coconuts and the gates of a wat. I walked through and found a small lake. From the old temple came the sound of monks chanting, while nearby was a great bodhi tree, with its leaves glistening in the sun. Further on, the size of letterboxes but ornately carved and elegant, were the spirit houses for the dead. They looked over the peaceful lake, the hills, and the rice fields, while the living transplanted rice seedlings.

On Thursday the 22nd July I was taken to Banteay Chhmar a temple, like the Bayon, that was built by Jayavarman V11 in the twelfth century. There were great tumbled blocks, tunnels, and towers overgrown by trees. A lot of the statues had been defaced.

As I walked back, I saw a wonderful face staring at me from a stone tower, full of gentleness, power, and love. This was Avalokiteshvara, the Buddha of compassion, also found at the Bayon. With such a Buddha and the resurgence of good monks I hoped, like Bob, the country would heal from the centre.

Edith, a blonde, slender Tasmanian in her mid-twenties arrived on Saturday 24th for a year and was based at the Ministry of the Environment. She liked the house and her room on top. Her boyfriend in Australia played soccer, and on Sunday she enjoyed watching a group of small boys playing while their cows watched from the sidelines.

The next day I worked on a proposal for the PAS members as the funds were inaccessible and we needed money to proceed. I had only seen 2 of the 8 PAS members deliver their programs. To Edith's delight, the PAS Education representative finally gave me back my motorbike. After his survey we decided to start with the three most challenging high schools, using strategies including drum groups and peer educators.

On Thursday 29th the NCHADS representative arrived. He was investigating the problem of AIDS patients selling their possessions and land for treatment.

A survey of 15,000 women in 2000 found that in Banteay Meanchey, the cost of one episode of transport and treatment for a health care episode cost on average $33, one tenth of the annual income. The money was commonly paid from savings (54%) or both interest and non-interest loans (20%). The Health Equity fund introduced in 2016 addressed the problem by providing free access to the poorest people for 2.6 million outpatient visits and 190,000 hospital visits annually.

I also met the local representative of UNICEF who took me to meet the Director of Education. The Director of Education asked us to hold HIV/AIDS awareness sessions with preschool teachers, and we did.

On Friday 30th of June, Edith and I went to Phnom Srok to see some of the 180 of the world's 1500 sarus cranes. They lived on a 100,000-hectare reservoir, Trapaing Thmar, where they were previously protected by conflict and landmines. When the villagers returned to farming they became vulnerable and the reservoir became a protected area in 1999.

Arriving in the afternoon we went for a walk in the village. This was former Khmer Rouge territory, and the village was wealthy with solid timber pole houses. Previously they'd made money from timber and now it was silk. We looked at the silkworms munching on mulberry leaves, then watched a woman weaving silk on a loom. People sat underneath their raised floors while ducks and chickens roamed around. This was another sign of both wealth and stability. When we returned, we walked upstairs to a big veranda crowded with hammocks and met the expatriate supervisor. From the veranda we watched the farmers tired and muddy, returning from the rice-fields with their hoes and metal rice caddies.

It took a while to fall asleep in the shifting hammock and I woke to lightening. Falling asleep again I awoke in the early dawn to the vibration of footsteps. Stiff and cold I climbed down the steep steps to the outhouse, the squat toilet and trough. There were ducks scrabbling for scraps, a rooster crowing and pigs in a nearby pen grunting. Already by 6:30 am people were walking out to the rice fields. The rains had come early, and they needed to plant. In the kitchen they cooked strips of pork on a couple of clay stoves fed with wood. A woman pounded herbs with a mortar and pestle. We ate rice and shredded pork and packed the remains for lunch.

It was now a perfect day and we drove out on motorbikes to the end of the track. After walking through water, then mud, we climbed onto a path. Walking towards the horizon in silence, the sky and clumps of trees were mirrored in the reservoir beside us. In front the Rangers chattered softly. They could read this place, where the fish would bite, whether it would rain and when the wind would change. At times they stopped to look at ants, beetles, and seabirds. Suddenly we stopped and the expatriate trained his binoculars on a distant group of trees. He passed them around and I saw the elegant white long-legged birds with their red cap.

When the sun was overhead, we stopped, and one of the rangers stripped to his shorts and began casting a net. A pile of small silver fish mounted up on the bank. Another lit a fire, another gathered wood, while another washed the rice. The small roasted fish were delicious, and we ate them whole.

When we got back, sunburnt, and tired, Edith and I walked to the giant ramparts of the dam and its gates. The reservoir was at least a kilometre square and from one to ten metres deep. As we looked over the vast expanse of water the water shimmered and the reeds shook, but beneath it was a sense of menace. This was despite the sand beach with gay little yachts, windsurfers, and kayaks. This reservoir was built during Pol Pot's time.

It was the last Saturday in June and we waited for transport. The CARERE expatriate engineer arrived with a sprained ankle after working on one of the bridges. He told me he wanted to replace as many of the wooden bridges as possible with concrete. He had seen many tractors bogged in the rice fields after the sudden rain caught them out.

Around six the truck which was to take us back still hadn't arrived. While the others swam, I sat on the reservoir wall, and watched a man poling a boat. I had enjoyed walking behind the four Khmer rangers. They told us 15 years ago 85% of this area was forest and there were more animals here than anywhere else outside Africa. In 2000 it was 1% forest and the animals had gone.

On Sunday we left in a pickup in the early morning after a noodle breakfast. We had to wait before a dismantled bridge. After we'd paid, they replaced the boards and we crossed. It would be more difficult when all the bridges were concrete.

I knew while I was at Phnom Srok, that hundreds, possibly thousands, had died building that reservoir. That was confirmed when I spoke with a Cambodian man who worked for CARE. He had been there. When he acknowledged this, tears filled his eyes, but he didn't speak of it further. He added he thought we were foolish wading through water where there could have been live mines.

———

On one of our trips the CARERE health officer told me about his time during the Pol Pot period of three years eight months and 21 days. He had ended up in a team digging reservoirs. He was eighteen when it began. When everyone was driven out of Phnom Pehn on 17th April 1975 he and his family went back to the village where they thought they'd be safer. They were grudgingly accepted. Things got tougher and more people were killed. He joined a band of sixty young people and escaped. They were caught and forty killed outright. Although he survived, he and his family were relocated to another village further from the border. Six of them were allocated one half cup of rice a day. They had to steal to survive.

He was then put into a mobile team, a team of young fit people which built dams. He had to move three cubic metres of earth a day. They woke at four am for study and then had twelve hours of work. At night there was more work, but many people could not see because of vitamin A deficiency or night blindness. To test for this, they pushed the person towards a latrine full of faeces.

If there was any hesitation that person was killed. Those who fell into the pit were relieved of their night duties.

I had felt the sense of menace that haunted that place as many Cambodians did. In the temples where many people were murdered, monks carried out cleansing rituals, but this was impossible everywhere. Those who survived were the young and the resilient and now they were in their thirties and forties. These were the people I was working alongside.

When we got back in early July, I got the worst diarrhoea I'd ever experienced. I woke in the night, during a storm, convinced warm water was dripping from the ceiling. It was my faeces slowly filling my pyjamas and then the bed. The smell convinced me. I hoisted myself up and hosed myself and everything down. Luckily the mattress wasn't affected.

A young woman turned up the next morning. How she knew I needed help I don't know, but it was such a relief to see her. She put the mattress out to sun, washed the sheets, hung them out, mopped the floor and then brought everything back in before it rained. Then, lying on the sofa she slept. The next day I felt better and read all day. I decided it was giardia and started myself on treatment. I also contacted my family, and we decided I would return for Christmas.

On Saturday we had dinner with employees from the Norwegian People's Alliance. They planned to take Edith, my housemate, to a border village where they were resettling 85 families on land the government had given them. But the military kept forcing them off, alleging they would cut the trees. Edith was to do an environmental impact assessment.

Poipet was also very unsettled. A sudden court judgement forced 955 families off their land and gave them two weeks to get out. This deadline was advertised on cable TV, which many didn't have access to. The military evacuated them. Many families disappeared, but 80 shifted onto land that had not been demined and one person lost a leg. Even the Governor seemed embarrassed by it. Corinne from ZOA was supporting them and I would go back when I was more robust.

Meanwhile I got proposals for the border areas and high-risk groups ready to take to Phnom Penh by September. Many people were helping. A former monk wanted to take 15 of the most senior monks in the province to check enlightened Thai monasteries. There was also a woman developing committees for old people in villages so they could be supported to look after their grandchildren if they were orphaned.

I began meeting the Director of Health each fortnight and submitted a work plan and report. He advised when Eap was to accompany me. Eap and I worked well together. He was connected to NCHADS, and the local Governors and Deputies. We also co-chaired the AIDS Technical Working Group.

On Wednesday I said goodbye to Sarin who had another job. Sopheak, her young niece who had trained with her in Phnom Penh, would work with me. First, however I would travel to a Thailand to learn about one of their temple-based AIDS Care programs.

Chapter Six

AIDS ZOO AND ANOTHER EPICENTRE
BOUENG TRAKOUN – JULY

I was on a bus with 45 volunteers from a Thai border village bound for Pra Baht Nam Phu or the Temple of AIDS in Lopburi on Thursday the 13th of July. It was a five-hour drive. Accompanying me was a Thai nurse from a hospital in Aran. The Thais wanted Thais in border villages to speak with Cambodians about AIDS and this was part of their education.

After lunch we drove up a valley with forest and large Buddhas on either side and pulled into a carpark alongside five other buses. We walked into a large assembly hall with a cloying sweet formalin smell, joining four to five hundred other people waiting. On stage was a huge heap of canvas sacks. A monk announced these were uncollected AIDS patients' bones. Clearly their cremation process wasn't as effective as ours.

Buddhists meditate on death and there was an opportunity to do this in the next room where bodies floated in formalin in large glass tanks. My companion saw a baby floating, while I glimpsed the flat yellow soles of its mother's feet pressed against the glass. We quickly withdrew and went to the next room, where there were more sacks of bones. We fortified ourselves at the café, surrounded by tourists licking ice-creams and drinking cokes before taking a hospital tour. That was even more confronting.

The nurses' station was glassed off, and the nurses stood behind it, natty in their white uniforms and starched caps. In narrow rows, in iron beds, skeletal figures lay, men almost indistinguishable from women, wearing just diapers. Wandering down the rows were tourists with small cartons of milk. I gave my carton of milk to a young, I suspected, girl.

"Peace," I said.

The only attendant at the bedside in that room of sixty patients was a white bearded man massaging a patient. The patient was frail and the massage vigorous. As I passed, I heard the click of the patient's neck. The white man looked up and we talked. He was thin but not emaciated. I wasn't surprised when he told me he had HIV and had been on antiretrovirals for over ten years. Many of these people, mostly under 30, were admitted after an accident and a routine HIV test. If they were positive and their family rejected them, they came here.

Looking at the sad young faces of those infected with HIV standing at the side, I knew time and hope had stopped for them. They helped care for and cook for these patients knowing this would be their fate. After leaving I told my companion I'd rather die alone in the rice fields like the Cambodians.

The following year I spoke with Graham Fordham, a social anthropologist who had lived and worked in Thailand for ten years. He said Thais could be cruel to those who were sick. In some communities, lepers had been put in cages. This was partly because of karma, the belief that the suffering of one's present life was caused by misdeeds during previous ones.

We were blessed with the monks and the leadership of the Venerable Muny Vansaveth. By the end of 2003 he aimed to have visited all 3000 monks in the Battambang area. The monks were provided with basic training about HIV/AIDS so they could provide education, care, and support in their communities.

On Friday the 14th I met Edith in Poipet, and we went to visit ZOA. Corinne, the Director, and I, went out in the morning to some of the settlement areas to deliver HIV/AIDS awareness sessions. We also answered questions about dengue.

In the afternoon we drove out to the site 10 km out of town where 80 families had been relocated by the military. Over 800 families had disappeared and there were still another 147 families waiting to be allocated land. The road was one of the worst I had been on, with the land cruiser up to its axles in mud. We stopped to pull out another car. It would be impossible to commute with the Poipet township by motorbike in the rainy season and many of these people worked there. We passed some pitiful heaps of thatch, and a few planks. These were the houses that had been dismantled, then left by the government authorities just a few kilometres short of the relocation site.

When we arrived, Corinne was surprised at the progress they'd made in a week. The government had provided some canvas and most of the families were now under shelter. There were a few shops and one enterprising man had started a restaurant. People were eating rice from a rough wooden table. There was a private pharmacy run by a nurse and a video parlour. The problem was water. They had drilled 45 metres and found nothing. Another organisation, Lutheran World Services was coming in a few days and would drill down to 100 metres. There were no toilets, and they expected a cholera outbreak. We walked around gingerly, sticking to the paths, as the area had not been demined. As the paper reported one person had lost their leg. We spoke with one man with ten children who had been a daily labourer at the border, and now couldn't get to work.

On Tuesday 18th Sopheak and I worked together, but first she told me about herself. She was 18. In two years, when she was 20, her mother and aunt would find her a husband. Her father had died the previous year. The prospective husband would pay $US3000 and they would learn to like each other. While the man could choose who he married the woman could not. Half of Cambodian women were married by 20, and this had been the case for two decades. Eighty five percent were married by 25. I found this confronting, but these arranged marriages were generally successful. The rates of divorce were lower than Australia. They were higher when the women were over 25 when they married, when the man was unemployed or if the woman had a much higher educational status.

Sopheak also told me the very rich pay $US100,000 for a bride and could elope with their lover. This was also the case with the very poor. The cost of a bride for a farmer was two cows. She also said the problem with condoms was they were associated with brothels and shame. The survey of 15,000 women in 2000 bore this out with less than 1% of married women using them.

We attended a military workshop in Battambang. Her English was improving. I asked if she could help with the translation about sores on penises. She said she couldn't, but she assured me she could speak with boys her own age, and we decided she would support the Red Cross volunteers and work with schools.

—·—

On Friday 21st I met Eap and we tried to untangle the Provincial AIDS Secretariate money. Some had been spent, some was owed by the department, and some had been paid back. It was unfathomable and I gave up.

Edith got malaria. She was an old Asian hand and had had it before. She felt miserable, developed skin wheals and when she took chloroquine they went. I wondered if I should take malaria prophylaxis as there were plenty of mosquitoes but decided not to. Instead, we covered our water jars and burnt coils.

On Monday evening, 24th of July I was very tired. It was such a long day. Meeting, meeting, meeting and yet things seemed to be slowly moving. I continued to enjoy the small things – the foal trotting alongside the pony and smiling up at the driver who smiled back. The dog running alongside me in the morning. The small boy I bought bread from, and the woman who watched us.

Wednesday and I was up in Battambang- the sun warming me. It was good to be away from Banteay Meanchey, the front line. I felt I couldn't let my guard down for a moment. It was a pivotal time in a pivotal province. If Cambodians had not changed their risky sexual behaviour when they did, the HIV prevalence could have risen to between 10 to 15%, killing many thousands more people. These figures were based on the East West Centre's Asian Epidemic Model. Geoff Manthey was aware of this, and I sensed it.

In the grounds of the crumbling two storey mansion next door a man chopped wood. In this area behind trellis fences there were many well-meaning charitable organisations with their four-wheel drives and their staff. It was more comfortable than Sisophon.

First of August. First day of spring and spring for the project too. There was a new Director at Mongol Borei, and MSF had noted an increased interest from the Provincial Health Department.

Down the road in Sisaphon a Catholic priest lived in a tiny house he'd built. He was offended when I asked if it was him who held the street film shows attempting to convert people to Christianity. He was a big fair man, a French German from Alsace. He took in a monk and after six months the monk had STIs, and possibly HIV.

I liked the Catholics. They helped when we heard a group of Southern Baptists were telling dying AIDS patients that if they didn't convert to Christianity they would go to hell.

I was in Battambang again on Wednesday 2nd August for a

three-day cluster meeting. We had representatives from six provinces, six Provincial AIDS Committees and members from each of the six Provincial AIDS Secretariats. We had representatives from Pailin, a border province whose governor was a former Khmer Rouge general. He defected and was given a province by Prime Minister Hung Sen. There were also people from Oddar Meanchey, another former Khmer Rouge province, the province the CARERE Director had assisted. There were still no NGOs in Oddar Meanchey, while CARERE was beginning to open an office there.

The next day Thursday Geoff Manthey arrived for one day with the Secretary of State. He told me he wished there were at least three of me as I was moving things. It was difficult to tell in the thick of it, still I did feel things were changing. I was relieved we might get help for the police and military from FHI/IMPACT. The Provincial Health Department also planned to start hosting monthly meetings in Poipet, and some NGOs had expressed interest in attending.

On Friday I had an evening meal with the UNICEF representative and supported her with a proposal for a floating school on the Tonle Sap. She said the girls left school at 13 to get married. Many of them were Vietnamese. Teachers from Battambang paid $12 per month transport from their monthly $20 salary, for the 100km trip.

They slept in the classroom or temple for the week and returned to Battambang at weekends. UNICEF had agreed to build classrooms and teachers quarters and there would be an HIV/AIDS component. We considered lifejackets and teaching teachers how to drive boats.

I was out when two men from the Thma Puok District AIDS Office called into the CARERE Office in the first week of August. Their boss had suddenly left, and they needed help to complete a proposal. There were still funds from the previous year.

On Monday the 7th of August I went to the market and got into a taxi at 5am. An hour later it was finally full, and we left. In the back I sat next to a bony old woman who coughed incessantly. I was worried she had TB so insisted they wind the windows down.

We were dropped at a quiet market. Although it was barely ten some sellers had already left. I walked down the wide empty road, relieved nobody had tried to wrestle my bag off me or bustle me into a rest house. There were shabby wooden buildings on either side, none showing any signs of providing accommodation. Finally, I accosted a man wheeling a bicycle with a flat tyre. He pointed to a low white building with a garish Khmer sign. When I knocked, a woman emerged, peered at me suspiciously and showed me a small bedroom smelling of paint. Reshouldering my bag, I took the road to what I hoped was the hospital. I'd always been driven there.

The hospital had an unhurried air and consisted of low buildings circling a large dirt compound. Women were washing clothes under a tap, while others lounged in the shade. I climbed up to the smaller building labelled administration and walked through knocking on every door. It was ten thirty. The Director of CARERE had told them I was coming. Giving up I went outside and sat under a mango , next to a youth in a grubby leg cast and a very young girl suckling a baby.

Finally, a big MSF cruiser pulled up and the staff member escorted me into the administration building. He knocked loudly on the second door to the right and opened it. Two men drinking tea looked up startled. They said they would contact the two men.

The MSF staff member asked where I was staying and when I told him, said he'd come back and pick me up at five. Twenty minutes later, two men pulled up on motorbikes. The Director of the AIDS Office was a handsome open-faced man while his companion the deputy was smaller and thinner. From their stumbled introductions I gathered their English was on par with my Khmer.

The key was found, their office opened, and they propped open the sash window and dusted the table. The Director presented me with a thick sheath of papers. I sighed. It was an ambitious but vague proposal.

"No," I said firmly in Khmer.

They looked at me puzzled.

"No," I repeated and then tried, "brothel", with an enquiring look.

They giggled and when both said "Boeung Trakoun", I nodded. We headed out. Although it was only 5 kilometres away it took over an hour because the road was so terrible. It was a fresh morning, and the rice fields were luminous green. There were piles of wood stacked alongside the road and two women were sawing a huge log with a cross saw, one above the log, one below. A huge truck laden with logs passed us. All the sizeable trees had gone leaving stunted scrub.

We pulled up at our first health centre and met the young

chief of one of the nine surrounding villages. I asked him how many people there were with AIDS. He said what I thought was nineteen. They corrected me. Ninety! This was in an area of nine thousand people. It was the highest figure I'd heard. These were men, between twenty and thirty, soldiers or police, or labourers who worked in Thailand. He said there was no help. We talked about strategies, education, condoms, videos, and village training. Then we went a few kilometres to the health centre. It was just far enough from town so people couldn't get there. The nurses charged patients and were not pleased to see us.

It was 11:30 when we arrived at Boeung Trakoun. It was a border village, dusty, narrow mud streets, rough wooden shacks, smuggled goods for sale, and children, who looked about five, roaming the streets with lighters and sniffing glue. Adults were playing what looked like bingo, calling out numbers and slapping down counters. There were sex workers lounging in front of their brothels, numerous young men, three to a motorbike hooning around, drunk, or drugged. They leered at the sex workers, played snooker, or watched videos in cramped little rooms.

We sat down at the only decent restaurant and the director immediately fixed his two posters to either side of the door entering the karaoke room. They were better than the tattered pictures of semi naked women inside. Food kept appearing and as we finished the bowls were replenished. As usual I paid. At intervals there were great thuds. HALO, the demining organisation, was letting off mines. We'd finished eating and were politely picking our teeth with toothpicks, when a Thai general strode in. He was a tall, well-fed man. very arrogant.

He looked contemptuously at us, while behind came his camp followers, a few civilians, and military staff. We left to visit the sex workers.

On the way we passed a barber. He had a picture of Buddha in the forest hanging outside his shop and was a cheerful chap. Men talked with him and he was happy to chat with them about HIV/ AIDS. He said he could probably sell a few condoms.

We talked to one of the five private pharmacists. Some were nurses but this woman wasn't. She knew people who'd died of AIDS, but she didn't know what she used to treat sex workers with sexually transmitted diseases and didn't want to know. She wasn't interested in learning about HIV/AIDS. Brutally I pointed out that if most of her customers died, she'd lose her business. She wasn't concerned. Finally, I asked her if she had any children. She had a 20-year-old son, and he knew how to protect himself.

The sex workers were more forthcoming. However, their information could be unreliable, their age for instance, when they said they were 18 and looked 13. The brothel owner always said the clients used condoms, then informally we were told about men who tore the condoms off just before ejaculation. The girls told us they had up to 10 clients a day, over twice the average of Poipet sex workers. They waddled, probably because of untreated sexually transmitted diseases.

A couple of girls squabbled in the background. One young girl had drawn a moustache on herself, longing to be a man. Many were illiterate, lacked numeracy skills and remained in permanent debt to the brothel owner. Numeracy training was recommended by MSF but there was no MSF here. At one brothel there were huge pictures of tulips flowers and country lake scenes, a distraction from the old wooden walls and mud floor. The brothel owner was shocked when I told her around one third to one half of these border sex workers had HIV.

We then met a small scrawny tattooed policeman. Although he took bribes from those crossing the border and the brothel owners, my heart warmed to him. He had a boxing club with 20 boys aged between 10 and 20 training every night. They used to be a football team but were addicted to yama, so he formed the boxing club. He said they no longer took drugs, but he needed more boxing gloves and bags.

The last person we saw was a monk. On the way back we turned off the road towards a few dilapidated buildings on a clay patch. We walked over to the chief monk's house and found him lying on a hammock. He quickly put on an orange robe while we bowed. He was a pale, anxious young man. Despite my colleague's sales pitch he assured us he could do nothing for the 90 people dying outside his gate. Neither could he help with prevention. This was because people didn't respect them. I could understand why. As we left, we passed a few teenage monks smoking, and the others burst out laughing. MSF had collected blood from these monks a few weeks ago, their theory being that monks were sexually abstinent. My colleagues presumed he thought I'd come back to tell him he was HIV positive. I made a mental note to speak with MSF.

We spent the following two and a half days in that pokey little office. We could only keep one window open because they didn't want dust getting into the vaccination fridge. The sole window kept blowing shut until I propped it open with a broom. I bought food and we even ate in the office, foregoing the usual three-hour lunch break. We developed a plan, and before this we spoke with teachers.

We planned to see the Director of District Health the following day, with the proposal to be presented to a meeting of the District AIDS Committee the next week. They would do more survey work of the high-risk groups and areas over the following month and their findings would also be presented to the District Health Director.

This district was the worst I'd found, but we had a good team. The village chiefs, and even the brothel owners were concerned. The service providers were problematic, but then I'd only met one of the pharmacy owners. The barber and police chief were gems.

I was optimistic and looked forward to our work together. Meanwhile I needed some downtime, and that wasn't far away.

Chapter Seven

BROTHELS & 100% CONDOM PROGRAM – AUGUST TO SEPTEMBER 2000

It was the 12th of August, the second anniversary of my sister Sue's death and I spent it at Banteay Chhmar, the temple that, like the Bayon, was built by Jayavarman V11 in the twelfth century. I was with Edith and her friend and I felt Sue would have approved as she revered the Dalai Lama. It was a fine day. Despite the desecration from looting and raids by the Thais we disentangled the three layers of the temple, the bottom which had collapsed, the middle bas relief, and the top towers with Avalokiteshvara, the God of Compassion.

A fifteen-year-old boy guided me; pointing out the bas relief with the soldiers, the king, his wives, the elephants, monkeys, dancing girls, and the fish and birds; and with my Khmer I understood him. He was one of seven and had been raised by his mother, a widow who laundered clothes and sold goods in the market. His father, a soldier, had been killed seven years earlier. He and his twin went to school and when he left, he wanted to be a water carrier. He and his friends had eaten frogs for lunch, so to supplement this we gave them pineapple and biscuits.

The soldier guarding the site had been a monk at Angkor Wat but had left to get married. He showed me some Sanskrit writing in one of the tunnels and said they got around 15 visitors a month.

The following week I was in Battambang speaking with young women from a jute factory. They were vulnerable, because of their low wages and naivety. Many of them were country girls and they sometimes sold sex to supplement their incomes. They had a lot of questions. I left them at 10.30am. It was glorious. Free time, at least until the early afternoon. I had been working seven days a week and travelling.

My next meeting was with a group of teachers. We watched a sad moving Cambodian film about AIDS, which I had found very effective for raising awareness. I had copied it with my own money and was distributing it as widely as possible.

On Friday the 18th I went to see Sarin. She had been nauseous for two days and was wretched. She couldn't drink and couldn't sleep. She said she was five weeks pregnant but too afraid to go to the clinic in case they prescribed medication which could harm the baby. The following evening, I went again, and she was a little better. She'd had orange juice and bananas.

I didn't realise how dangerous it was having a baby in Cambodia, and I'm glad I didn't. Maternity related deaths were one of the leading causes of death for women between 15 and 49 years. In 2000, around 430 women out of 100,000 who gave birth, died. Most deaths were preventable. By comparison in Australia, between 2000 and 2002, the maternal mortality rate was 11.1 per

100,000 women. At least Sarin was a midwife and knew what she was facing. I hoped she would navigate the system safely.

The weekend towards the end of August was busy as I prepared to return to Phnom Penh with proposals. I spent Saturday translating questionnaires for Thma Puok, and spent Sunday with a Help Age representative. She believed Help Age could encourage villagers to raise funds for self-help groups through Old People's Associations. These groups could then fund loans and savings schemes to help the elderly care for their orphaned grandchildren. It was a clever idea and an important one. Visiting AIDS affected families I had often observed elderly parents caring for their children and grandchildren and this was confirmed by the statistics. The parent was the carer for 80% of adult AIDS patients and spent on average 7 months caring before their child died. Two thirds of grandparents supported their orphaned grandchildren and half of these did so, despite financial hardship.

There wasn't enough money in villages to generate funds for self-help groups, but from 2003 to 2007 Family Health International supported older carers and People living with AIDS (PLWHA) in 19 villages in Battambang. They did this through home-based care teams and Old People's Associations. The elderly carers and PLWHAs were supported with transport, low interest loans, tools and seeds, gifts of rice and assistance with raising cows. This support had a flow on effect, as the villagers learnt more about AIDS and supported those families affected by it.

The following Tuesday, 22nd August while waiting for Sopheak to translate the Provincial Profile, I ruminated on an accident I'd just had. I was carrying eggs on my lap on the motorbike and when I got to the gate, lost control of the accelerator. Thankfully Sopheak had opened it and I shot through, decelerated, and as the eggs fell off my lap, slowly fell over. I didn't hurt myself or the bike but cracked the eggs. I made an omelette, and we ate it immediately with fresh bread.

To divert myself I wrote about the downside of returning to Australia. How dull the roads would be. No potholes, no mud, no huge trucks suddenly stopping in front of me, no people riding on the wrong side of the roads, no children wobbling around on bicycles, no pony carts clopping along and obstructing everything else, and no heavily laden motorcycles with the driver straining to control the load. But this accident was due to my lack of skill and my inability to juggle eggs and ride a motorbike simultaneously.

On Sunday I walked over to see the children at the orphanage. Three young girls had arrived, the eldest fourteen. Their mother had died, and their father could no longer care for them. I gave them some books and asked the others to support them. As a solo parent I couldn't imagine what he went through. At least his daughters would be fed, educated, and have others to play with. The worst orphanages fed into sex traffickers and brothel owners, but I believed the Sisophon orphanage, with Sarin's husband involved, was not one of them.

Before going to Phnom Penh, I returned to Boeung Trakoun and enjoyed meeting the village chiefs, teachers, police, nurses, and monks. Someone else paid for the daily allowances and refreshments. This was most uncommon. We decided we needed to establish STI services, especially for the sex workers, provide peer educator programmes for the military, support the police boxing club and the barber, and work with the NGOs and village chiefs to get education to the general population. We were still unsure whether there were ninety cases out of nine thousand villagers, so the District Aids Director was doing a survey which I would check when I returned.

At the meeting we had a frank discussion about condoms. The chiefs told me men in the area didn't like using them, so I asked why. They said sometimes men were drunk or drugged with yama, and sometimes the sex workers complained because of irritation. My colleague from MSF promptly brought out a box of condoms which were super lubricated. The chiefs were impressed, and all tucked a few into their shirt pockets.

I had an unpleasant night at a guesthouse there. There were fleas in the mattress, and mouse and rat droppings. The water was very muddy, as were the sheets and towels. At midnight I sprayed myself with insect repellent and I slept after that.

Late in August I was back in Battambang talking with the military. They were underfunded and at risk. We needed to get IMPACT/FHI involved. The military and police fed into the high HIV prevalence rate with their sexual risk taking. The Behavioural Sentinel Surveys from 2000 showed that while most men had 9 lifetime partners the military had an average of 43. Rural police averaged 31 while urban police had 4 with the proximity of their families a major influence. Reported condom use with sex workers by the military was 70% in 2000. It was a shortcoming and needed to be dealt with quickly, and it was. With donor support, peer educator training and programs, and condom availability the rate of condom use with sex workers amongst the military rose by 16% to 86% in 2001.

I was impressed by the military hospital in Battambang where 15% of their patients had AIDS. The doctors cared and even paid for antibiotics to stop AIDs patients getting PCP or Pneumocystis Carinii. This Regional Military Hospital (Region 5) received support from June 2004 from the Ministry of National Defence, NCHADS and FHI.

I then attended a meeting of the Battambang Provincial AIDS group, and took their agenda, proposals, and questions to Phnom Penh.

———

I travelled to Phnom Penh on the last day of August through Pursat. I wanted to learn about their Provincial AIDS Committee, as I'd heard it was active. The Director had been invited to Japan for four weeks to present a country profile and develop a proposal for Japanese Aid. Pursat was the third largest city in Cambodia and bordered a large river. Like Battambang it was peaceful with large trees, good roads and quietly decaying French houses, with huge verandas, airy rooms, and wooden floors.

On arrival I met the AusAID consultant working on sexual trafficking with the Ministry of Women's Affairs. We got on well and travelled together to Kampong Chhnang the next day, a fishing port on the Tonle Sap, just a couple of hours from Phnom Penh. It was good to have a break before I arrived in Phnom Penh. We had a party, but it was difficult for me to switch off. There were many people from Phnom Penh and some back packers. I returned to the house around 11. At 2am they let off some firecrackers and the police turned up thinking it was a shoot-out.

In Phnom Penh I spoke with World Education, about incorporating HIV/AIDS awareness into their programs. World Education, an international NGO, worked in schools, educating teachers and children about land mines. They spent a month in each area and UNICEF had asked they include an HIV/AIDs component. They were willing to come to both Battambang and Banteay Meanchey Provinces. I subsequently met up with them in Pailin and Malai, two former Khmer Rouge Provinces.

I learnt the 100% condom programme would be implemented in Battambang and Banteay Meanchey provinces within a couple of weeks. I also found some good interactive videos, some for schoolchildren, and others targeted at beer and dancing girls. Videos were good for those with poor literacy skills.

I needed a break so went to Sihanoukville for a few days. This coincided with the two weeks reflection time before the public holiday celebrating the Festival of the Dead. Monks around the country were preparing spiritually, as Christians did for Lent. Legend had it that during Jayavarman VII's time a monk came back from hell unscathed at this time and said the dead could be freed from suffering if they were remembered.

On the way down in the bus to Sihanoukville on the 9th of September I was thrilled when we drove past a range of hills, high, steep and still forested. I talked with the young engineer beside me who worked at the Sihanoukville port which received one million tons of cargo a year, largely cement and construction materials. We passed large plantations of bananas and cashew nuts owned by Generals. The land grab by the military was something I had discussed with the previous Australian Carere Provincial Director who was now based in Phnom Penh. Following Pol Pot many were operating in survival mode, grabbing what they could when they could. Long term goals and the common good were not considered.

I arrived at Sihanoukville that evening to find two large frigate birds flying into the wind with large, white forked tails. They cruise the currents in stormy weather and reminded me of the Solomons, where I cut my teeth on intractable problems. After marrying a Solomon Island journalist in the mid-seventies, I worked as a nurse and a journalist for seven years. It was raining and there was a line of forlorn shelters on the beach with hills behind.

The next morning it was fine, and I went for a swim at six. The water was warm, and I surfed on the small waves and stood letting rivulets of water drag the sand from beneath my toes. A woman searched the beach with two small boys in grubby clothes. A couple dragged a net in a semi- circle pulled it to shore and suddenly dropped both ends. They both ran to the flopping in the water and the tiny fish. Even here there were little sparrows in cages beside the restaurant.

In the evening, I went down to the little shelters to buy a beer and watch the sun set over the sea. The five boys in the room opposite mine, invited me to dinner. Three of them came from Sisophon and one was in his third year at medical school. He was raised by his mother, a tailor, and now an uncle in the States was supporting him through medical school. It took 7 years and he wanted to be a paediatrician. The three other young men had completed year 12 last year and the last was studying computers.

We talked about many things, how many siblings they had (mostly 4 to 6), why there weren't any dolphins here, generally about my work, whether there were many girls studying at university (not many), about sports and how they were missing their mothers (they were). Their mothers were about the same age as me. They took pictures and we vowed to meet tomorrow. Two had never seen the sea before and thought it was wonderful. As we were talking the next evening a young man, about their age appeared out of the dark with a sack on his back. They threw him a couple of cans and he disappeared.

I was back in Sisophon on Friday, and as I listened to music I felt I had turned a corner. I no longer felt I was trying to clean the Aegean stables. Others were assuming responsibilities, the gates were opening, and the donors coming.

Sarin was admitted to a clinic for three days for vomiting and given four types of medication. According to a nurse from MSF there were two she shouldn't have had. I asked Sopheak not to speak to her about it as I didn't want her worrying about it for the rest of her pregnancy. It was awful having her on that narrow veranda above the jail while she was so weak. Her sister-in-law locked her in when she went to the market, and people brought her food. She couldn't eat most of it including grapes.

The next day, Saturday, I went to see her again. She looked a little better and was eating seasoned porridge. Sopheak's mother was there, and they planned a memorial ceremony for her husband, who died a year ago. She had a soft, delicate, sad face and looked at me wistfully. Sopheak was different, tougher, perhaps like her father. Sarin wanted a cotton dress, so I gave her the cotton I'd bought for my mother.

In the afternoon I went to see the orphans. They were swimming in a muddy dam, in what looked like an old quarry. I perched on the red clay soil at the side. They were splashing, laughing, and clambering on each other's backs. Some could swim. The fourteen-year-old girl I'd befriended, the oldest of three sisters, got out early, dried herself and showed me a picture she had drawn of a goose flying above the sun. I gave her a simple book and she read it to me falteringly. She couldn't read English at all when she arrived a few weeks ago. She was learning fast.

———·———

The day after I left to attend the demonstration 100% condom program in Sihanoukville. I'd just arrived back from Phnom Penh two days before, but I was booked to fly from Battambang beside one of the MSF nurses who had flown just once before. I woke at 3.30am to barking dogs and chanting monks, took the truck to Battambang and boarded the plane with the MSF nurse. She sat tensed and tight lipped until we finally emerged above the clouds, then looking down, said they were pretty.

At the bus station we met Corinne from ZOA and two more staff from MSF. Corinne took a taxi from Poipet, a 12-hour journey, as it was cheaper than an airfare. My companion from MSF was delighted to see the sea. She'd never seen it before.

Corinne and I stayed at the rest house I'd been at a few days earlier while the others went to a more expensive hotel. We went swimming and I raced some small local boys who could barely swim but beat me anyway. That night we looked up at the biggest star, Kai Chao. On the horizon were fishing boats attracting the fish with bright lights.

On Monday we woke to a grey dawn and a half-moon, preah kai. People were fishing in the pink flush of sunrise. The sea was flat, and on the beach were numerous heaps, of krill, tiny fish which had been dredged with nets. By doing this I suspected they were cutting into the fish stocks but there was little consideration of sustainability because people were too desperate. Just out from shore boats were looking for kai, about the size of a spectacle case.

That morning, we went to see a posh brothel run by a Vietnamese with 27 sex workers. We climbed to the top floor and looked over the sea. The MSF nurse from Phnom Penh said the Vietnamese were preferred because they were paler, had better hygiene and were better educated. They were also more expensive.

The brothels down by the port were very different. There were rows of them marked with red paint and the police kept a record of the girls, including photos. Sometimes relatives came and collected them but for many there was no other option. In 1998 there were 60 brothels in Sihanoukville with 500 brothel-based sex workers and 200 entertainment workers. Socially marketed condoms were available in the brothels and sex workers attended STI clinics monthly for checkups. A condom use working group and outreach team worked with local authorities and brothel owners and implemented the program. The Vice Governor was head of the Condom Monitoring and Evaluation Committee.

A MSF worker from Phnom Penh supported the Cambodian Prostitutes Union. It was founded by Tia, a 28-year-old woman, forced into prostitution after she fled an abusive relationship. Two weeks after she began, she was badly beaten by a client and felt completely alone. She founded the union in January 1999, and it attracted 200 members. The Director of the Cambodia Women's Development Association was impressed and supported them financially and administratively. Each Friday morning, they met, talked, and learnt about HIV transmission. Client violence, worker safety, and health care were discussed together with human rights. Members distributed HIV brochures to their colleagues..

Dyna, one of the members, gave a very moving speech at the first National Conference on Gender and Development on Sept 7th 1999. She explained she was not garbage but a sister, a daughter, a person, someone who was trafficked, raped, beaten, and forced to accept men for sex. Every day she endured humiliation, harassment from the police who locked up sex-workers with no bread or water, then sold them to a new brothel for $US100. They had to pay the police and authorities bribes to continue working, and they were in bondage to the brothel owners. If the client paid an extra fee to the brothel owner, he did not have to wear a condom. Dyna called for recognition, human rights, and punishment for those who infringed them. Their union survived.

On Wednesday the 20th September we boarded the bus for Phnom Penh and passed an accident. A car had gone through a fence and there was a big oil tanker off the road. A woman's body was laid out on the verge, her face covered. Life was so precarious. But it was time to return to Sisophon for the Festival of the Dead, which despite its sombre title was a celebration.

Chapter Eight

PAILIN AND THE KHMER ROUGE
– OCTOBER 2000

Cambodia has more festivals than anywhere else in the world, and it was now Pchum Ben, the Festival of the Dead. Everyone went home for the fifteenth day, and I was no exception. I arrived back in Sisophon on Thursday 21st of September, the day before the public holiday. It is believed that the dead become ghosts, and to avoid angry ancestors the living need to honour them.

It was good to be back, and I walked to the rice plains. There were boats on the river and many huts were surrounded by water. Ducks, pigs, puppies, cows, donkeys, and drunken men celebrated, watched by silent women. The occasional flags fluttered in the fields to scare the birds away from the ripening grain. The wind furrowed the rice and blew on the great flat elephantlike leaves of the lilies. Then there was an unearthly twanging. Someone had unwound a cassette along the road and a man was strumming the tape.

The great rain clouds hung above the plains, white bottomed, with thunderous tops. The distant trees were inky. A storm was coming. Yes, I was meant to be here. Synchronicity as Jung called it or the universe in alignment. I read a lot of Jung in my adolescence and even bought *'Dreams, Memories, Reflections* with my Grandparent's birthday money. My grandmother wasn't impressed, although she too was Viennese.

Yes, the universe was so much larger than we commonly acknowledged. Some Cambodians felt it too. Like Sopheap, the CARERE religious affairs officer and former monk who told me in a pagoda he had known me in a previous life. I thought it quite reasonable, as it would account for that extraordinary dream which brought me over.

The next day, Friday, was the public holiday and I knew exactly what to do. I got up early and cooked food for the monks and biscuits for the children. I packed the food and my wat clothes, and I took the road to the wat in the caves outside Sisophon. The road was deserted, and I walked past yellow jute flowers and a cow herder sitting in a tree resting.

At the bottom of the steps to the wat I bought a coconut, then sat on a bench under the mangoes to drink it and change into my wat dress. A woman talked loudly to herself, and they told me in Khmer it was because she was 'old.' After climbing up I went inside.

An old monk lay on his bed. He took my food, my incense and my candles and he prayed with me. I prayed for the dead including my brother and sister, and all those who had died and would die in this country. I thought of the Buddha, the great King. who abandoned it all to search for enlightenment.

How simple things were, how little was needed and yet we in the West worshipped consumerism. It was so good to be in another culture, the better to see one's own. As an eleven-year-old in NZ I'd befriended a Cook Islander, and helped her to boil the greens, or puha, and look after the baby. Again, my grandmother complained. I overheard her speaking with my parents, but they said I should be left alone.

I took the biscuits to the orphans, and on arrival sat on the veranda watching 15 children drawing. The others had gone home to their families. They had such imagination. They drew hills, elephants, fishes, and suns with faces. One drew a patchwork of fields, with flowers, trees and tree stumps, roads and people walking along them. Another drew a dragon flying, a man on his back. Some pictures of people were almost Picasso like, simple and clear eyed. Then they drew ice-creams because they were hungry. When they left for lunch, I went home and saw cows in Sisophon for the first time. They were having a holiday too. The cow herders rested while their cows picked at the rice-straw haystacks.

In the afternoon I walked out to the rice fields. Some of the rice was beginning to ripen and there were white scarecrows to frighten away the birds. Many of the huts were marooned, with ducks dabbling around them, and sometimes a boat was moored beside the road. A thin legged, broad-shouldered Khmer strode along the road with a large pestle, while his naked infant son ran behind him. A man swooped down blocking the child from his father, and the boy cried. His father turned, smiling.

There were drunken men driving a tractor up and down the road, while men daubed with charcoal branches around their head danced. One man quietly threw up beside the road. The women watched. Men were drinking rice wine, cheap and plentiful. Occasionally they included pesticide to make it tastier and somebody died.

The women watched because when the men were drunk there could be fights and violence, with women coerced into sex without condoms. It was a risky time. One third of women with no education or primary education had experienced violence in the previous 12 months from their husbands. This dropped to 12 percent for women with secondary or higher education.

I was back in Battambang on Sunday ready to leave for Pailin in the afternoon. I had stayed overnight with a friend and in the morning went for a run.

A small girl with an old sack on her back searched the rubbish bins in front of each shop and pulled out a piece of string from the bin in front of a money changer. The money changer ignored her. Further on I passed three mannequins, one very white, one very green and one, a male, with an Akubra hat. Suddenly I noticed three Khmer men, as still as the mannequins staring at me.

Later I went to a bar and tried to watch the last day of the Sydney Olympics. The connection was poor, so giving up I walked to the rice plains. I sniffed the salty air, while a boy fished, and others flew kites. Far off was a military base, a wooden gabled building with flags flying. I passed a soldier's hut on a corner. It was tiny, not much higher than chest height, and the sides were open. Inside was his mosquito net, two rifles and his military khakis. He was cooking on a few embers in a big pot, his floor a piece of corrugated iron.

There were children everywhere, skipping, flying kites, and sliding jandals along the road. The older boys were racing on motorbikes. I thought of the Buddha I saw in Australia in an art exhibition before I came. Buddha was cracked and old, but around him the green of new rice was sprouting.

———

I'd been invited to Pailin at one of the Provincial meetings. It was a former Khmer Rouge area, 80 km from Battambang and 20 km from the Thai Border. There were brothels outside Pailin town, and at the Thai border. In 1999 the HIV Surveillance Study (HSS) showed from 10 to 25% of the brothel-based sex workers were HIV positive. The virus was also crossing into the general population. The prevalence in antenatal women below 30 was 2.3%, while antenatal women above 30 had a rate of 4.5%. No wonder the women were angry and closed one of the brothels.

Although it was just 80 km from Battambang it was a gruelling three-hour journey. It was a moonscape, the forest gone, but as we got closer there was jungle on the hills. The driver told me the Khmer Rouge decided not to log these trees. Perhaps it was also because this area was one of the most heavily mined on earth. We drove past a hill which looked like a ship with a big monastery on top. Further along, on a hill shaped like a crocodile, the driver said there was a nunnery. The nuns cared for women who had been rescued from brothels and got leftover food from monks. There were upland rice fields, browner than the flooded lowland rice, and crops of yellow flowers, jute.

The driver told me he'd worked in the border camps in public health, and they had treated STIs and undertaken contact tracing.

Finding work was difficult now, he had five children and had to bribe people to get work. I asked him why so many Khmer men went to brothels. He said before Pol Pot few men went because it was shameful, and they lost face. But after Pol Pot it expressed their freedom. Again, like the generals and their landgrabs, they were in survival mode and lived for the moment. He didn't think the 100% condom use policy would work because of alcohol and drug affected clients. The sex workers moved every three months because clients got bored with them.

He also told me traditional birth attendants did abortions. A survey of 15,000 women in 2000 found in Pailin ten percent of women had abortions compared to 1 to 3% in other provinces, with most performed before the fourth month of pregnancy. While 60 percent of abortions were performed in a health facility the other third were performed in homes by traditional birth attendants. Their clients were at risk from sepsis and tetanus, and sometimes died. Sex workers were also at risk with one quarter having at least one abortion, while less than 5 percent using contraception.

The driver dropped me at the guest house, and I walked around the town. I was surprised at the wide streets, but the two storey buildings were beginning to deteriorate. The grandest building, the Provincial Governor's Office looked like the hotel in Sisophon we called the Wedding Cake. Nearby were small offices with signs, Tourism, Energy, Rural Development and Mines. Three years earlier in 1997, Ieng Sary a former Khmer Rouge Commander, met Prime Minister Hun Sen and Pailin became a municipality. There were no schools, and people were illiterate as they'd been fighting most of their lives. There were few laws.

Leaving the centre of town, I walked to the market where people were weighing gold. Rubies sold for $100 and small blue sapphires for less. It was quiet and no one seemed concerned about security. Rubies, sapphires, and timber exported to Thailand maintained the economy for many years.

It was strange weather, and the hills were covered with dark rain clouds. I walked up to the temple, Wat Khaong Kang built by migrants from Burma, the Kola or Kula people in 1942. During the Khmer Rouge period many fled to Thailand, others were used as labour in the mines, and some killed.

As light rain fell, I studied the churning of the ocean of the milk. It is a scene from Hindu mythology with demons holding the king of the serpents by the head, while the gods hold him by the tail. During the churning of the ocean of milk many treasures are pulled up, including the moon, the asparas and some goddesses. There was one old monk, and I felt the sadness, the brokenness of all that had happened here. Before the altar were three candles burning in a boat. I prayed and was graced by a sense of calm and hope.

I then walked to the other temple Phnom Yat, also built by the Burmese migrants. It was brightly painted, and I felt less comfortable, so I left and sat beside a stupa, a mound containing the bones of monks and nuns. Sitting alongside the stupa, under a gnarled old tree, I looked across at the patches on the hills and wondered if that was where the Thais had mined. Unlike the Khmers they had machinery.

The stupa was erected in the honour of Yiey Yat Yat, a sorceress who warned the Kola to stop killing her animals. She said when they stopped hunting, they would be rewarded. They went into the jungle and saw an otter playing near a stream and when the otter opened his mouth, it was full of jewels. The jewels were still there and when it rained heavily the villagers came to look for them, as they washed down the gravel road. Back at the guest house I ate on the balcony overlooking the lights on the hills, wondering if they were huts, although I hadn't noticed them during the day.

I was busy over the next few days touring the hospital, clinics, and nearby brothels. On Wednesday October 4, back at the guesthouse for lunch, I scribbled a few notes as the rain drummed on the roof. I'd spent the morning with the Department of Health and there was stream of people. The X Ray machine didn't work. There was no time to write a report, but I noted that Provincial AIDS Secretariate meetings needed funding, possibly from the World Bank.

I'd seen the World Education man, and we'd been out together. They had some very poor communities where the children were naked and didn't have enough to eat.

I also visited the border crossing and the Flamingo Casino with its seedy karaoke bars. I liked the Khmer women who travelled with me. They were strong, independent and forthright.

On my last day I went back to the temple. A motor taxi driver practicing his English told me there was a lot of malaria here, and a man working here for three years got it four times. He said malaria had become treatment resistant and he was right. By 2016 the multi-drug resistant malaria strain from Pailin threatened to derail malaria treatment throughout the world and kill millions of people. The deadly plasmodium falciparum had become resistant, not only to Artemisinin but to its partner drug Piperaquine. This was because of the casual way untrained people distributed treatment, and the lack of control by the authorities. In 2019 WHO carried out a mass drug administration in the area and everyone was given treatment at the same time. This dropped the incidence of malaria in the population in that area from 77.8 per 1000 in 2000 to 5.8 per 1000 in 2020.

At my farewell dinner with the Deputy Governor, we were served roasted wild birds. I couldn't eat them.

On Friday night, the driver returned to drive me back. It was the only time I was ever driven in a car in rural Cambodia at night as it was too dangerous. It was ironic that the only safe route was from a former Khmer Rouge outpost to Battambang. We finally left at 4pm on the terrible road and although I was jolted continually for four hours, I enjoyed it. We were thrilled when at sunset, we saw a deer. People sat outside their houses talking, after their animals had been gathered into small sheds. Later as the night came, they lit smoky fires to keep the mosquitoes away. Across the rice fields I saw the flickering blue light of a TV. It was a village closer to Battambang and more prosperous.

The driver told me he hoped to settle in Pailin and set up a business because it was semi-autonomous and close to Thailand. He spoke longingly of Thailand, of the stability, the lack of corruption and the strong opposition.

I didn't go back to Pailin. I saw no need to. I met the Director of Health the following April and he told me they had an NGO arriving, had funds for the Provincial AIDS Secretariate and were beginning the 100% condom program.

In 2000 the Lonely Planet said there was little point going to Pailin unless you liked hanging out with geriatrics responsible for mass murder. In the recent edition they spoke of the two wats and a pleasant waterfall. Pailin has also grown. In 2000 there were 3000 people in Pailin town and 8000 people in the province. In 2023 there were almost ten times that number; 79,000 people in the province.

Once the mines were removed the province boomed. I was not surprised. There was discipline, gender equality and less corruption. Malai has also done well. In a conversation I had with a UNHCR officer she said people in Pailin were afraid to commit crimes. When I was there, there wasn't a jail, and while there were police, they weren't visible.

———

When I returned to Sisophon in mid-October, I joined another Provincial AIDS Secretariate (PAS) workshop and found a vast improvement. The emphasis had changed from talks in villages to educating ministry staff. The PAS members were interested and absorbed and understood the importance of their role.

I also wrote to my family:

Things are moving fast. The Health Department has swung around and is working with NGOs and districts. NGOs are getting more money and support from donors. The World Bank has come through with a strict auditing process.

We have a sound connection with NCHADS in Phnom Penh, and Eap, the Director of the AIDS Program and the doctor who is the Provincial Director of Health, and I work well together. If there are any concerns, we check with Phnom Penh.

The district hospital improved after they changed the Director. He is a decent guy and is getting help from the World Bank. He wants me to go down in a couple of weeks.

The border areas are slowly getting attention. Poipet is still a worry, but FHI, a big NGO is starting to work there. We are getting together a proposal for the other difficult border district Thma Puok which includes Boeun Trakoun and it is likely to get money next year.

And I wrote to my son John, hoping it would arrive for his nineteenth birthday on 16th October.

Happy Birthday. I hope you have a lovely day. I'm very much looking forward to seeing you all again.

Everything OK here. It has been raining for four days. As soon as you step out of the gate you are swimming in mud. There are streams running down the roads and you find on a motorbike the mud comes up to your thighs.

I keep going. I love the countryside and the rice fields. Some of the rice is almost ready for harvest and yesterday I walked past a big field where the grains are now yellow. There were rags strung around it and men banging drums and shouting sporadically at the circling birds.

On the 2nd November I wrote in my diary about my deteriorating mental state. Finally, the pace had caught up with me. I was exhausted and not sleeping well. This was how Cambodia was for me, great highs and great lows. I was witnessing unavoidable death and suffering on a major scale, and yet there was also the touchstone of the deep spirituality I found in this country, the beauty of its people and the land. But it was tenuous and there was the constant risk of burnout and even collapse. Underneath lay my homesickness and the certainty that my nuclear family, myself and my sons, had irreversibly broken up. Again, I wrote in my diary.

It's been a while since I wrote. Lot of stress. Haven't been sleeping well.

I went up to Battambang and then went out to see Arlys who was on holiday. We discussed education workshops and the agenda for the first working group meeting in Battambang. It should be OK.

But the rest of the morning was nightmarish. I was driving along the road on the bike, hit a big rut and my purse flew out. I picked it up and went on, then returned after realising my house keys were missing.

Had to buy new ones in Sisophon. I was stopped by the police going around the roundabout the wrong way and fined. Refused to pay. Then had to get back to Battambang for meetings. Felt sick. Came back and went to bed. Finally had a good night's sleep,

Went to meeting with the Thais, including one woman I met on the bus to the temple. They think things are working better now. Told them we were planning to start soon in Boeung Trakoun. Had lunch together. They were teasing the Director of Health about learning Thai. He is more relaxed, even jolly now.

On Friday 3rd November I spent the whole day of slogging over proposals. Lost my voice.

By Monday 6th I had lost my voice again. On the back of a pickup. Hemmed in from every side. Put a cloth over my head and resigned myself to the dust. Here in Cambodia a dog sits in the middle of the road and the traffic goes around it.

I hear Dad's doing a locum in Coff's Harbour. How I long to see them again.

Chapter Nine

FAMILY TRAGEDY, TOURING, HOME FOR XMAS – NOVEMBER TO JANUARY 2001

A friend of my son John died by suicide on October 30th and my oldest son Brian emailed me on the 7th of November. He had been drinking and took the train home. After being fined for not having a ticket he lay down on the track in front of the next train. That afternoon Brian went with John to the scene, which Brian said was a mistake. They laid flowers nearby and went to his funeral. His family were distraught. It was completely unexpected. John was living with his girlfriend's family, and they were very supportive. I felt I should leave and tried to call from Sisophon but couldn't. John emailed me on 9th of November and said he couldn't understand it. I left that day for Phnom Penh and like John, kept wondering why it happened.

I got to Battambang on the 9th on the back of a pickup and stayed the night with Arlys. She and her American friends were watching the election Bush vs Gore and there was no outcome that night. After speaking with her I realised if I could, I should stay another six months to stabilise the gains we had made.

On the 10th of November I went down to the marketplace to get a taxi to Phnom Penh and waited for an hour. The driver was an excitable man who was about to leave when the police came and took his keys. Another driver turned up, a good one. It was better than flying because it calmed me and connected me with the countryside. It was a lovely day, the sky washed clean, and I had the front seat to myself. While some of the rice had been ruined by the floods, in others it was heavy with yellow ears, and in others it had been harvested and laid out to dry.

These floods in September 2000 affected more than 1.5 million people and killed 179. The damage caused to infrastructure and crops reached $US 50 million. There was still water lying around and little boys beckoned us through the crossings. Generous passengers gave them money and we also stopped constantly as they gave money to the women sweeping the road.

I could have gone straight through to Phnom Penh, but I was afraid of the thousands of extra people crowding the city for the water festival. I was tired and fragile, so I got off at Kompong Chhnang just 90 km from Phnom Penh. I walked to the markets, bought a sandwich, then sat near the Tonle Sap. Rested I took refuge in my room, a white painted cave with forest green curtains.

In the morning, I ran around a track in a school ground where boys were playing soccer and girls chatting. Curious, I took a path to a huge derelict building which I discovered was a rotting stadium. What glory days were those? Now there were cows grazing in it. Continuing along a path behind it I stumbled on a guard post manned by demobilised soldiers and retreated. At the market I squashed myself into a taxi. It wasn't far, but it was slow, and there were numerous roadblocks. Close to Phnom Penh we were directed through the back streets.

I stayed with my friends, a volunteer couple. We checked the time difference and I decided to ring in the evening. Meanwhile we went to the waterfront where there were a million extra people. Trucks were busing people, standing in the trays. On the river-bank food was prepared in woks, bigger than any I'd ever seen before. We shook hands with a gorilla, and there were condom promotion stalls.

The canoes started racing, two heats at a time. In some boats they stood and paddled using their oars. These were faster than the long elegant 60 seaters, with a bosun in front. I enjoyed watching the men with mallets, knocking various parts of the boats. They were maintenance men, like the mechanics in the pits at the Grand Prix. In the evening there were fireworks, and the trees were alive with fairy lights.

I got through to Dad, who was very happy to hear from me. I then spoke with Brian who said I was to finish what I had started. John wasn't there but I called later and was very relieved to get him. He was OK. He had a good job and was saving for a car. He was interested in photojournalism and had sold an article for $200. It was such a relief to speak with him and he asked when I'd be coming home.

"Christmas," I said.

On Monday I was down at the waterfront again, and my hosts had gone to work. More racing and another lovely day so I decided to follow the crowds and walked back to the hotel. While I waited for the AusAID consultant, I laid down on the sweet short grass and looked up at the sky. There was no short, sweet grass in Sisophon. She arrived and we went inside. She had lost weight and was in a stylish blue trouser suit. The hotel was elegant, simple, and beautifully proportioned and she said it was the nicest hotel she'd stayed in. We had a drink in the elephant bar, browsed in the very expensive shops and then lazily swam up and down their pool. She was tired and said sexual trafficking was difficult because there were so many vested interests.

I also visited a few night clubs with a friend. It was fun and I could finally tell my teenage sons I'd visited a nightclub, and not for work either.

At the first nightclub there was middle aged European sitting at the bar, having his shoulders massaged by a young Khmer girl. I gave him a contemptuous look and wove past to collect a free Phnom Penh Post. I learnt he was the editor.

Later the Nestle man turned up and we had a very jolly conversation about the ethics of promoting bottle feeding in a developing country. It's not promoted by WHO because infants are likely to die from contaminated water. The Nestle man assured us he promoted breast feeding so the journalist offered him a two-page spread. He discussed using the stone breasts of the elegant woman dancers engraved on the temples to do so.

We ended up at the Heart of Darkness. This was interesting with snakes in bottles, spiders, bats hanging from the wall and an out of place replica of the Statue of Liberty. The seventies rock music was a break from the high mincing voices of female Khmer singers.

Who was there? Everyone who didn't fit anywhere else. Gay people, drug addicts and volunteers. At least it was a break from middle aged European men and young Khmer girls.

On Tuesday, the 14th of November, the Chinese President Jiang Zemin visited Phnom Penh. It was historic, as no Chinese President had visited since 1963. Mao had supported the Khmer Rouge.

The city was clean and for the first time I saw rubbish bins in the streets. There were huge posters of the Cambodian King and Queen alongside posters of the President of China and his wife. School children lined the route waving flags of both countries, and there were banners across the road reading 'long live Cambodia.' It was a fruitful visit and cemented a close and ongoing relationship. China agreed to give Cambodia $US12 million in grant aid and loans and offered help to flood victims.

I decided to go for a brief break before returning to Sisophon and I'm glad I did. I didn't get another chance to visit the Bokor Hill Station and Kep, places I found both haunting and evocative. Bokor Hill Station encapsulates Cambodia's history as nowhere else. but anyone interested needs to get there quickly. The Chinese plan to swamp the site with luxury houses, a casino, a hotel, and a luxury go kart track.

On the 15th November I left early. It was to 150 km to Kampot, and 37 km up to the Bokor Hill Station.

It's early and I'm sitting in a minibus writing and waiting to go to Kampot. A child selling bottles of water and chewing gum is watching intently. Someone has sat down behind me and poked a long stick through which gets in the way of my feet. A small smelly child and her father have sat down beside me. The child outside is watching me sadly.

We leave and I have time to inspect the slender man beside me. The baby is about the size of a newborn but is probably six months old and smells of stale urine. A very docile baby the father says, as he amuses himself with a small plastic spoon. His father shades the baby from the sun with his hat and then puts him between his legs. But the baby doesn't appear to like that. He is almost limp and lacks muscle tone.

The rice fields on the way down have not been affected by the flooding. This is fertile land, and the town is known for its fruit, its pepper and its durians. A river runs through the town, which reminds me of Battambang with its terrace shops. There are also old colonial houses, some abandoned.

I booked into a guest house and immediately hired a motor bike taxi to take me up to the Bokor Hill fort. The driver and I started climbing the less fertile foothills of the long snakelike forested range. The road was rough and the going slow as we were on a 100cc bike. He drove well and had an air pump and his tools strapped to his front mudguard. We stopped while I paid a $5 entrance fee, and I heard an eerie noise like that of high fretsaw. I looked up and saw a flash like a cuckoo.

The driver told me there were elephants and tigers, but he'd never seen them. Although it was a national park, some trees had been cut and sold by the army to Thailand. Around a bend we came on people squatting and eating out of pots and plates. Further up there were little shacks and plantations with people selling pineapples, bananas and jackfruit and hens. We stopped for lunch and ate bread, fish and the fruit I'd just bought. The bread was very good, soft and crusty. We passed the black lodge of King Sihanoukville.

Finally, at 2pm we arrived at a clearing. In front was the ocean, and above us racing clouds. It was cold, and often windy and misty, with mist from the west. The motorbike chain had fallen off and as the driver fixed it, I watched a hummingbird hovering over the flowers and flowering vegetables. The sun was brilliant, unrestrained, falling on the leaves and breaking them into thousands of shimmering dots, like an impressionist painting.

We got back on the bike and passed black angular rocks, in which I found heavy sculptured faces. Then we reached the top and pulled up in front of the crumbling Bokor Palace Hotel. It was such a haunted place, overlooking the escarpment, the sea far below. I could imagine ruined gamblers hurling themselves over the cliffs. It had solid external stairs to the balconies, perhaps for illicit liaisons, or to escape from fires.

The French colonialists built it in 1925, or more accurately, it was built by indentured Khmer labourers 1000 of whom lost their lives. It was a settlement with a villa, church and previously a post office and was abandoned by the French in the late 1940s. In 1953 they were defeated by Ho Chi Minh in Vietnam, left the region and Cambodia became a monarchy. Bokor Hill Station flourished as the playground for wealthy Khmers in the fifties and sixties, but the Khmer Rouge gained more territory. In 1972 the hill station was abandoned for the second time.

Although the Vietnamese took Phnom Penh in 1979, Bokor Hill fort remained a Khmer Rouge stronghold. There was fierce fighting for months in the 1990s with the Vietnamese in the hotel and the Khmer Rouge sheltering in the solid Catholic Church. Both were riddled with bullet holes. The church was empty apart from the altar and on entering I thought how strange it was that it had provided a haven for the Khmer Rouge.

The US didn't have the same concerns about the Khmer Rouge as I did. They supported them during the eighties with military training, preferring them to the Soviet backed Vietnamese and denied the genocide taking place during Pol Pot's era. I am grateful I didn't know this when I was there.

Coming back through the forest in the late afternoon, I took off my helmet as I wanted to absorb the smells and sounds and sight of that forest. There was an offering on a stone wall to the spirits, some bananas, and pineapples. The Chinese don't have the same respect for the forest as those who left offerings at the wall. Instead, they have a 99-year lease and plans to obliterate it with luxury houses.

From Kampot I got a motorbike taxi and went to Kep 20km away, and just 30 km away from the Vietnamese border. We passed through salt mines to salt marshes, where fishing boats were drawn up beside houses squatting over the water. People with nets fished from wide bellied, elegantly carved boats. They were Muslims and the women wore head coverings. We passed women cutting and binding rice into bundles, with rice drying by the side of the road. There were graves in the rice fields, and shacks. My driver told me that in Vietnam they grew two to three rice crops a year compared to Cambodia's one.

Then we arrived at the sea and Kep with its crumbling French colonial mansions. Kep was destroyed during the fighting between the Vietnamese and the Khmer Rouge. In 2000 it was not a popular destination because electricity was only available five hours at night. It was quiet when we arrived in the morning. The sea was blue, the sun played on the gentle waves, there were islands in the bay, and mangroves. We drove past the promenade towards the King's house, now open, and I wandered through a few of its huge rooms, cautiously because it was used as a toilet.

We went down to the jetty where a little boat with an engine pulled in. There was a pile of tiny fish and another sackful drying on the jetty, used for duck-feed. The only living things visible were a few crabs in the mud. Closer to town trucks arrived with people standing on the back. Some were monks who had come to study, while others had come to enjoy themselves with their female companions. I was told it was also a refuge for those who couldn't find work or didn't want to. Sometimes garment workers from Phnom Penh came to make extra money selling sex.

I went for a lazy swim and watched the insects, and the swallows which swooped down on them. I doused myself with fresh water which cost 1000 reil, then ate cassava-coconut pudding and sesame cakes, and went for a walk. After discovering a white elephant cave, I noticed a stupa nearby. Unusually it had a door, so I went in.

Behind an altar was a dying Buddha, while above him a Khmer Buddha floated, an angel attending him. Buddha was dying and I thought of my talk with Arlys. She was right. It was critical to consolidate what we had already done. My family understood I needed to come back.

On the 27th November I returned to Phnom Penh and stayed with my friend the AusAID consultant in a hotel overlooking the Mekong. Each morning, I walked beside it and watched the sunrise. In the evening, we went to the Foreign Correspondents club, a fascinating place. We chatted for three days and then I caught a taxi back to Battambang. By late November the proposals for Battambang had been submitted and I returned to Sisophon.

Eap told me we needed to begin working with the local NGOs, and I agreed. I tidied the house and packed. Edith had left for a homelier and more private place in Sisophon.

On the 2nd of December on the way to Poipet, I was crammed in the back of a taxi, while the woman in front effortlessly and almost soundlessly, vomited into plastic bags and threw them out the window. I distracted myself by looking at the green and yellow heads of rice mixed with the white plumes of other grasses. I never tired of the rice-plains. In Poipet I made my way through the beggars and then negotiated the cost of passage with the border guards.

In Thailand I finally relaxed and made my way to my friend, Corinne's house. We ate at the night stalls, and the next day I spent swimming and marvelling at the quiet calm prosperity of the Thais. I bought apples at the market and gave one to a stooped old monk who blessed me. There were no money changers in the street, instead I had to go to the bank with my passport.

On the 3rd of December I slept well for the first time in months. The pressure, the responsibility was lifting, at least until I returned. Finally on the 5th of December I flew home from Bangkok.

Chapter Ten

WORKING WITH NGOS AND BEGINNING SITUATION ANALYSIS – JANUARY 2001

It was such a relief to find the boys were alright when I arrived back in Brisbane. John had borrowed money for a car and had two part-time jobs, while Brian was waiting to hear the outcome of his application for an IT degree at QUT in 2001. It was good to be back at Cedar Creek for Xmas, swimming in the creek and climbing up to the waterfall. On 6th Jan Mum took me back to the airport.

When I crossed into Cambodia and took a taxi, I found the rice harvest had begun. In the distance I saw a tractor and behind it, rice stalks blown in the air. Everywhere there were rice stacks like Van Gough's haystacks. Beside the road children tried to poke fruit off a tree with a pole. In Sisophon I took a pony cart to the house. Opening it, I found everything covered with a fine layer of dust with boot prints through it.

On Monday when I woke at six it was still dark. In Brisbane

in summer, it was light by then. My new guard Bo had left. He worked as a motorbike taxi driver or motordop during the day. I ran up the laterite road, the red sun squeezing over the hills. It was so dry the bones of the hills at the end of the road were showing, the trees in the little orchard looked dead, and the grass between them had withered. On my way to the market, I found a couple more brick buildings had gone up while I was away. My language had lapsed but I made myself understood and bought pegs, lotuses, and food. On my return I cleaned the altar, lit the candles and incense, and put lotuses in a vase. The house was alive again. I gave money to a young monk, and he blessed me.

It was good to see my language teacher in the evening. I had to start at the beginning again. The demining company he worked for CMAC had stopped while the donors audited their finances. He was back teaching Grade 12 in the morning and private students in the afternoon.

On Tuesday I saw a large, armoured tank with heavy wheels, a few portholes in front, and heavy steel shutters. They were deminers from the HALO Trust, Norwegians, and they had a sauna which Edith was later invited to, although I suspect she never went. HALO had been based in Cambodia since 1991, when they began clearing mines to ensure Cambodians could safely return from the border camps in Thailand. By 2016, their 25th anniversary, they had cleared half a million landmines from the country. With the other demining agency CMAC, they were on track to achieve Cambodia's goal to be free of landmines by 2025. HALO also employed men and women from the communities they worked in, boosting local economies.

Another interesting sight was the motorbike assembled from spare parts. It was driven by a rakish looking man towing a small-covered cart, selling cooked chickens. Best avoided I decided.

I went to see Sarin. She told me they thought she might have placenta praevia, or the growth of the placenta in front of the vagina. When the vagina dilated, the placenta could bleed putting the baby at risk. She was crocheting and afraid to travel on bumpy roads. This was a gruelling pregnancy and she said it would be her last. Sopheak was there and we left together. The sky was dark, but Sopheak assured me it wouldn't rain. It was a slow start to the year, and I was enjoying it.

Edith returned looking happy and relaxed on Wednesday the 10th of January. She had visited her office at the Department of the Environment and found the desks dusty. She suspected no one had been there since she left. Eap was also back. He said he had missed me, and I was told to be at work by 8am on Thursday. Talking with Bo that evening I learnt there had been an eclipse the night before. He said that during an eclipse Khmers ate lots of fruit. It seemed odd and I suspected there was a communication gap.

On Thursday afternoon I realised why I'd been told to come early that day. It was a roller coaster. First, I learnt from AusAID that none of my proposals for the Provincial AIDS Secretariate (PAS) had been accepted. Then we found the World Bank wouldn't give money for the PAS and NCHADS could only offer training assistance. I saw Edith briefly and told her I felt like leaving. Instead, I visited some local NGOs and found they were having an NGO forum the next day. Then I rang up a colleague about the PAS who said the Asian Development Bank might be interested.

Eap was pleased. He said work was easier when I was around. Arlys also invited us to a meeting at the training centre. This was the beginning of the provincial situation analysis with the final product delivered to NCHADS in July that year.

In the evening there were less mosquitoes and I enjoyed cooking and Bo's company. My language teacher described him as a slow learner, but most people were, compared to him. I was. I went to sleep dreaming of the face of compassion, the Avalokiteshvara,

On Friday in darkness, I ran up the laterite road, towards the hills and the moon. The two geese that had hissed at me a couple of days earlier ignored me. I passed a small baby lying on a table next to the loaves the mother was making. Wrapped in a piece of calico the baby smiled blissfully at the universe. It was just 6, the lights of motor bikes cut through the darkness, and people were walking to the market. A sudden gasp of happiness took my breath away. Cambodia was like that. It had been a peaceful country before the American bombing and the rise of Pol Pot and sometimes I had glimpses of that.

That morning, I attended the NGO forum and learnt about their programs. Some organisations were happy to integrate HIV/AIDS into their work and some had already done so. The KBA (Khmer Buddhist Association) representative said he provided home care to 19 people living with AIDS (PLWHA) and their families and had two PLWHA as volunteer speakers. They provided practical support including rice supplementation. They also supported people to access hospitals and clinics and 20 orphans in villages.

They did excellent work and were the one of two Cambodian

NGOs included in a regional UN report featuring HIV/AIDS initiatives. They began HIV/AIDS prevention activities in 1997 with sex workers, brothel owners, uniformed personnel and out of school youth. In 1999 they also began to provide care and support for PLWHA and their families, and orphans. Some organisations worked in schools, and we discussed the possibility of PLWHAs providing sessions.

Back at the house in the evening I looked out the window at the dusty banana leaves. Just one week ago I was in Australia with the family, as we ate a meal together. I hoped it would be easier this year.

The next afternoon I met the Director of Health. He wanted me to focus on cross border issues and he wanted the 100% condom program established throughout the province. He had been reconfirmed in his post which I was grateful for. He told me we now had World Bank money for the 100% condom program, with CARERE prepared to give us $10,000, and UNICEF filling the gaps. It was also possible the Asian Development Bank would support the PAS program. We discussed whether AIDS patients could be nursed separately. In Thailand the monk's AIDS hospital was one of the most depressing I'd seen, and I said this. When antiretrovirals were available, People lived with AIDS rather than died, but at that stage they were still very expensive. They were available privately for US$250 to $US280 per month but there was no guarantee they were not fakes. Not only patients, but nurses and doctors felt the situation was hopeless.

It was still dark on Saturday when I left for my run, and I passed the forlorn form of small boy clutching a blanket. There was another with a great sack on his back, making his way to one of the recycling houses, while another hauled a trailer with a great stack of flattened cardboard cartons. He shouted imploringly to his friends.

Later that day Edith came around. She'd decided to keep a pet lizard. It hid in her bedroom and woke her every two hours throughout the night with its calls. We walked through the rice fields. The rice has been cut and laid out to dry. In some areas, near water, they were ploughing with oxen. I had never seen the rivers so low. On the muddy banks they had planted rows of vegetables. On the river men were fishing from their elegant, keeled boats.

We sat down at a little stall near the river and bought a soft drink. Walking together through the laneway of trees I was grateful for the shade, but Edith said they were acacias, foreign trees which stopped the growth of the natives. Part of the rice canal was bright green with algae. Back at home we ate delicate little eggy pancakes, filled with beansprouts, lettuce, cucumber, and tomato. We dipped them in satay sauce. I asked Edith about nightclubs. I thought women took their clothes off, but they didn't. Khmer men didn't tolerate women taking their clothes off in public and yet sixty percent of them went to brothels.

On Sunday, we went to see the orphans on the motorbike, Edith was rather uncomfortable sitting on the back with a heavy bag. It was good to see the 14-year- old girl I'd been supporting. She was becoming more confident and had her tiny 13-year-old sister with her. With the children we went back to the temple in the limestone cave. At the entrance there was a monkey tied to a rope. We followed the limestone steps into the bowels of the mountain, into the large grotto.

The old man was there with a woman making decorations for the altar. It was more elaborate than I remembered. A serpent's tail curled around on the rim of an oblong concrete water trough. On a raised platform was a substantial double bed with canvas strung above it to stop the bat droppings. In silence we bowed to the altar. The old man and woman took little notice, except the old man muttered a few words about not being able to speak with us. I realised he had broken his vow of celibacy and was embarrassed.

My 14-year-old friend decided we should leave and led us back. At the top the monkey had escaped and was being chased by two young monks. They had wound their yellow robes around their waists and tucked them up like shorts. The children threw stones at the monkey trying to coax it towards the monks. Instead, it turned and ran towards us. The more threatened and frightened it was, the more aggressive it became. I was worried it had rabies. Some children ran, and it chased them. Some children stayed still as I asked them to. I left a gap and allowed it to escape.

Then we walked home. There was a pretty, dead, black and white patterned snake on the road. The hills were so dry they looked almost burnt. We passed the lake where I had floated flowers for John's friend. It was lower and partly covered with algae, but still beautiful. A kingfisher perched on its pockmarked mud banks. We passed boys who threw crackers at us despite my protests. Two small children sitting beside the road on a rug were having a picnic. It still felt like a holiday.

I went to sleep late on Monday night. I was lonely and missed my family. Now Edith had moved, I needed to rent out the top floor. After making this decision I finally fell asleep clutching a piece of blackened wood from Mt Barney near Brisbane.

———

It was very cool on Tuesday, a golden morning, then it clouded over. Edith had flown to Phnom Penh. I had two separate meetings with NGOs. Both were working well, had good leadership, and wanted to integrate HIV/AIDS awareness into their programs. I spoke with a representative from World Education Cambodia. They were carrying out mine education in schools in heavily mined areas including Malai. I had seen their work in Pailin. In Malai they held a four-day training session for head teachers and teachers. The teachers spoke with the children, and they went home and asked their parents questions such as was there a risk because children played with landmines, or was it because adults cleared the land with knives? Was it both? The children then drew, created role plays and songs; and a concert and exhibition were held for their parents. World Education worked with parent committees and wanted to integrate HIV/AIDS awareness. We agreed to meet in Malai.

I went to see an officer from World Vision about the sponsorship of one of the orphans and he told me that during a home invasion his 17-year-old-daughter had been shot and killed.

Very sad. Violence lurks just below the surface as the Australian High Commissioner warned us.

On Thursday evening the 19th of January Bo told me his 73-year-old stepbrother had just died. Bo, who was in his early thirties, had been raised by an elder sister after his parents died. Bo told me he'd missed me and asked why I couldn't live in Cambodia. "Because my family in Australia would miss me, just like your family would miss you if you lived apart from them," I replied. Then I remembered both his parents were dead.

My language teacher and I discussed the various words for caves, including a cave for animals, or a cave in a mountain. We talked about the serpent's tail I had seen in the cave temple. The serpent is a dragon which guards and protects. We talked about my altar, and he said it was traditional for Cambodians to burn 5 sticks of incense together to keep away evil spirits. Then I asked him about the spirit houses at Thma Puok. He said after Pol Pot few people had them. He also told me there were very few native Cambodians left, just a few in Ratanakiri. Most people had intermarried with Chinese.

On Friday after my run, I had a leisurely start. As there was no-one in the top floor, I sat on the balcony eating my porridge in the soft early light. First it was apricot, then pearly white and then grey. Peace. I looked down on a fine middle-aged man with greying hair in a pony cart and he looked up, slightly ashamed. I noticed his left leg below the knee had gone, and he was holding the stump with one hand and the reins in the other. The little boy who slept in the hammock under a tarp on the verge in front was still asleep. His boots were still there, carefully laced up.

Then the problems of the oncoming day began to flood in. My computer had stopped which meant I had to work in the computer centre near the bookshop where there weren't viruses. The motorbike had stopped too, and I was worried it couldn't be repaired. Talking with my language teacher that evening I told him about my bike and how I'd been walking all day. He said he found too much walking difficult. After walking around with the deminers for three days he got burnt and his face peeled. One of them told him to go and sit in the car. He couldn't drink like the Europeans either as his face got spotty.

The following Thursday I was up in Battambang and tired. The daily round had caught up with me. There was a loud wedding less than a block away and the Green Parrot had changed its name to White Rose, although it made no difference to the food. It was still fried rice, but I couldn't be bothered going anywhere else. That was a shame, because I'd had good meals in Battambang.

I'd spent the morning with one of the Doctors . I was stunned by the difference. When I'd first me him last year he refused to speak English, or even hear it and blinked incessantly. Now he no longer blinked, and his English was good. He had presence and confidence and presented me with a very comprehensive and well thought out plan. He wanted help with the border districts and wanted me to come every month. Then I spoke with one of the senior doctors who had been a great support. Sadly, he was leaving Battambang in February, but I asked if he could come back every three months to help with proposals.

It was the end of the week, and I was drinking down at the river with NGO workers. They told me a story about two girls enticed from their families in Kampong Cham who ended up in Battambang where middlemen tried to sell them to brothels. They would only take one and said the 15-year-old was too black and ugly. She found her way to the police station, the Human Rights NGO and then the UNHCR officer, who got her back to her family. They couldn't tell me what happened to her sister. One of the big problems was ignorance. Only 10 percent of women in Banteay Meanchey had heard about the law against sexual trafficking while it was over one half nationally.

Back in Sisophon on Sunday I was disorientated. I slept soundly and woke up at what I thought was six. I jumped out of bed and rushed outside. Bo was still in his hammock with a mosquito net over him, and surprised. However, he got up and took the net down, meekly folded it away, then got on his motorbike and left. It was dark, with a crescent moon. There were very few motorbikes around. I made my way to the street where I run. There was a truck depot with overnight lighting, and I ran up and down in its beam, the upper boundary defined by a pair of barking dogs. The sky wasn't getting any lighter when I left, and I couldn't understand why the market was still in darkness. When I got home, I realised it was six.

We had a housewarming party on Sunday night, at the UNHCR Officer's house. She had been in Cambodia for four years, three years in Siem Reap and one year in Sisophon. I asked her about Corinne's concerns in Poipet.

ZOA supported four villages on the border. When the commune officials asked for numbers ZOA refused to provide them. Thirty-four people some very senior, disputed the villagers right to live on the land they were occupying, and planned to take the case to court. The UN Human Rights Officer said the villagers were advised to get a legal representative. Minor officials then visited them and said if they did, their lives would be in danger. A special envoy from the UN would visit Poipet in March to assess the land issue. She also said the commune elections had been postponed for 2001. I was relieved as I had experienced riots in the Solomons during elections and knew that time could be volatile in Cambodia too. It was time to get back to Thma Puok where the villagers were at risk, not from the authorities but a virus.

Chapter Eleven

CHINESE NEW YEAR
– FEBRUARY 2001

Travelling to Thma Puok on Monday 22nd January, the driver took the new laterite road built by CARERE. As I looked down on the brown stubble of the rice fields, I saw women collecting sugar palm leaves to shore up their roofs while men dug in the mud for fish. There were other men swinging water in a bucket from one level to a higher one. It would be two or three months before it rained.

After calling in at the MSF health centre we drove to the hospital. In the long low timber building, with its rows of beds inside, there were patients with pneumonia, beriberi, and many with TB. In 2002 Cambodia had one of the highest TB prevalence rates in the world with more than 1500 cases per 100,000 people. By comparison Australia in 2001 had 5.1 cases per 100,000 people.

In 2001 a survey found that 64% of Cambodians were infected with the TB bacteria but not all had symptoms. There were signs of it everywhere, the people in taxis who coughed incessantly, the spit on the ground in the markets, on the paths and the hawking. What tipped people into showing active symptoms was often malnourishment. In 2002 almost one quarter of the population or 23.6% was malnourished. By 2021 that had dropped to 6%.

The country used the WHO recommended DOTS (Directly Observed-Short Course) six-month treatment. The use of multiple drugs and the observation of their administration guarded against resistance developing. At the Thma Puok hospital, TB sputum positive cases were admitted for the first two months, then treatment supervised at clinics for the last four. The doctor said after five months of treatment patients were generally sputum negative.

When people were infected with HIV their immunity dropped and they were more vulnerable to TB. HIV prevalence among TB patients increased from 2.5% in 1995 to 10% in 2005. When antiretrovirals were available, patients coinfected with HIV and TB received treatment for both, with the timing depending on the patient's condition.

During the ward round at the Thma Puok hospital we also saw a boy with a cleft palate, open almost to his nose. He was referred to Phnom Penh. The doctor said she had referred six during the previous year. In the Thma Puok town I had seen a child with no nose, and another with a large growth between their eyes. The doctor said there were three with facial abnormalities.

When I discussed this with Edith, she said there was a BBC team in Poipet investigating a Thai company who sold toxic agricultural products to Cambodia. A recent study confirms there is an association between the exposure of fathers to pesticides and the higher incidence of cleft palates in their children.

Around 5pm I walked along the dusty road to the dam. On either side were timber and thatched huts and alongside them great heaps of rice straw and husks. Ox carts passed, loaded with bags of rice. A man pushed a cart loaded with large black plastic jerry cans and children. Everyone, biking, walking or on motor bikes, carried large black containers. They filled these from the two large square muddy dams in front of the wat, tied them to their carts, bicycles and motorbikes and left. I was told this water was for washing. The drinking water was collected when it rained, and stored in large clay water jars which had to last through the dry.

One in ten children in Cambodia died before their first birthday with major childhood illnesses including diarrhoea, fever and respiratory infections. A survey in 2000 of 15,000 women showed in Banteay Meanchey 20 % of children under five had diarrhoea in the previous fortnight. During the dry almost one third of rural woman in Cambodia had to get water from rivers and streams, lakes, and ponds.

Walking back, I met the Deputy Director of the District AIDS Office, who introduced me to his wife and their 15-month son. He had built his own home for $US5000. It was on stilts, with several bedrooms and a veranda He also worked as a photographer to supplement his US$20 monthly government salary. He told me they had engaged a woman with a motorbike to do the condom selling. All three of them were booked to attend a three-day workshop in Sisophon about condom selling, and financial and project management.

Back at the house I went to a party in a hangar, a previous UNTAC canteen. I played ping pong with the doctor and talked with a guard who was trying to learn English. His wife had died of AIDS, and he had a six- year-old daughter.

At another party back in Sisophon I met the Agricultural Advisor from AusAID. He had finally taken the train from Pursat to Battambang. It left at 1.30pm and got in six hours later. His advice was to take the first carriage as even the second had a one metre sway. People rode on the roof. I'd seen them as I looked across the plain from the taxis I travelled in, watching the train snaking along with tiny figures sitting on the roof. In Battambang a man and woman leapt for the train, the man clinging to safety, the woman falling. She was crushed. There was also a shoot-out with police pursuing people on the roof.

He also told me five deminers working for CMAC, out of a group of 70, were HIV positive. He asked about condoms, and I told him about Population Services International or PSI. PSI was established in Cambodia in 1993 and launched a social market condom for Number One Condoms which are still widely used. They have provided over 9 million condoms. The deminers were another high-risk group, and like the military worked in border areas and were away from their families for extended periods. I discussed it with Eap and advised the Director of Health and NCHADS.

Chinese New Year began on the 23rd of January and for a couple of days beforehand there were small boys letting off crackers in the street, some as loud as a gun shot. Edith had some thrown at her in the market. On the 23rd the sun was orange with the fine dust of the dry rising with the cracker smoke. I celebrated by placing a beautiful pink rose from my garden on my altar and lighting 5 incense sticks. Mozart's flute concerto competed with the mayhem outside.

Edith and I went to Sopheak's for lunch. We had roast chicken and pork, some nice dipping sauce, vegetables, rice then puddings. We watched a famous opera, about a beautiful Khmer woman engaged to a rich man, but in love with a poor man. It ended tragically. The rich man killed the poor man, and the young woman killed herself. At Sarin's house there was a carpet of red banger shreds in front of the door. The table was laden with candles, fruit, biscuits, and goblets of tea. I danced around with a sparkler.

On Wednesday the 24th the volleys of fireworks started at 5am, just before the wat bells and then came speeches over a loudspeaker for a funeral. I fled to my hill, avoiding groups of small boys. The sky was pink. A couple of older boys wheeled out a double amputee in a three-wheeler chair, a small wheel in front, to watch me. When he thought I'd gone he laughed. I was glad I had given him pleasure.

Later we left on motorbikes for Mongol Borei and I had Sopheak's sister on the back. We turned off and followed the Rohatuk River, with its riverbanks terraced with vegetables. There were big trees and big houses, many of them owned by overseas Chinese. When we arrived, we went to watch a dragon fending of a man in a red mask with a sword. Back at the house we ate warm curried chicken and I walked down to the river and sat watching the women casting their small fishing nets. A farmer sat down beside me and asked if I had a husband. Caught off guard I said no, so a girl sitting nearby suggested I marry him. I left and back at the house helped the girls carry our plates down to the muddy river to wash them.

The next day Thursday, the 25th at 6am, the crackers up started again but I couldn't go for a run. I had diarrhoea and had been up four or five times overnight. I was grateful it wasn't worse. As a former health inspector, I knew the perils, and also knew there was no way to avoid it if I wanted to participate in family gatherings. I hoped my gut would toughen up.

———·——

My language teacher was adamant, when we met on Friday evening, that men could not sexually love their wives. That would spoil their life together and wives were not to express sexual pleasure. It was only the West that believed in romantic love and marriage. A girl was expected to repel a boy's advances and they did. A survey from 2000 showed that Khmer women usually married at 20, with almost 90% virgins at the time of marriage.

He added, the virgin or possibly widow, had to have a good character. Men tried different sexual positions particularly with Vietnamese, but not with their wives. If a man was absent for a long time, it was understood the wife could take another husband. My language tutor loved his wife and had obtained her parent's permission to marry her. When I met Geoff Manthey the UNAIDS Director, he confirmed this. Khmer men didn't expect their wives to pleasure them and would be very suspicious if they did.

My language tutor was late the following Monday evening 29th January, as he stayed with Bo and watched a red glow on the horizon. Across the road a truck took off. They had gone to help their relatives knowing there would be no assistance from the authorities. Twenty-five houses on the road to Battambang were on fire. Every year in Sisophon there were fires; sometimes caused by the misuse of gas, sometimes by faulty wiring, and sometimes arson. The Governor didn't have a fire service and the police, who used to have a couple of trucks, had sold them.

The next day I met the Thma Puok doctor in Sisophon. She was upset about a girl bitten by a snake who had been sent home. When she returned, she was dying. The doctor would have sent her straight to Phnom Penh for anti-venom.

That day Edith told me about an accident she had seen. A taxi went past at great speed and outside the police station, clipped a man on a motorbike with his wife and two children. The man flew off the bike, hit his head on the road and Edith heard the crack of his leg breaking. His wife was distraught, but the children were alright. The motor bike taxi drivers rallied around the family while the police pursued the taxi. Edith kept going as we were advised to do by the High Commissioner.

I also received an email from Community AID Abroad advising me of a position in the Solomons for a community development officer. The Solomons was imploding. Much more than a Community Development Officer was needed. In the end it took RAMSI, the Regional Assistance Mission to Solomon Islands, and 3 billion dollars. The next day when I went to the Provincial AIDS Office, I was exhausted and upset about the Solomons. I would return but on my own terms and when it was stable.

On the first of February, Thursday there was a ceremony for the Director of Health. I distinguished myself by being late. I had left in tatty trousers and returned when I realised I'd have to wear a skirt. I jammed myself into one and rushed down. One of the ladies couldn't bear my dishevelled look so when I entered, she led me out and pulling and pushing straightened me up. The men watched from the side windows. I was led back in, to the broad grins of everyone including the Governor.

The Governor was good looking and mild, with two determined deputies who continued writing during his speech. The guests were seated according to seniority with Eap and I halfway down the table, MSF were closer to the front and the Director of CARERE closer still. The Thais were in suits and there was talk of fixing problems and good work.

We went to the restaurant at 11am, the women in elaborate silk dresses. Again, we were ranked according to seniority. The women sat together except for me and the female representatives from MSF. The karaoke was very loud and various people sang including the Director of the PAO from Pailin. I asked the MSF doctor why it was so loud, and she said most people had recurrent ear infections as a child and many were deaf.

Friday was spent at a farmer's field school in Sisophon providing HIV/AIDS awareness. Edith was there too and was amazed at what they learnt about including soil fertility, companion planting, and the safe use of pesticides. They were starting from a slow base with poor yields, caused by their lack of knowledge about the application of fertilisers and pesticides, poor soil, poorly prepared fields and poor irrigation. Once they corrected these problems their yields increased, and they used less seed. The rice straw which the cows fed on was left in the fields to increase fertility.

On Sunday, 4th Feb I went by taxi to Battambang. Staying with a volunteer friend I listened to the chanting monks, the fan and the whine of an occasional mosquito. It was hot on my mattress on the floor. I was still sweating from my afternoon walk. I had gone to check on the demobilised soldier who lived on a little bamboo platform on a back road. He made a living, or tried to, by stopping trucks. He had a large bamboo pole. I watched a truck approach but as he lowered the pole it reversed.

On Monday I had a meeting with one of the District AIDS Officers. There has been a problem in Kamrieng a commune in Battambang bordering Thailand. One of the NGO officers paid the health staff to carry out HIV/AIDS awareness with motor bike taxi drivers. This took the nurse away from the health centre. Because of their poor pay they needed these extra allowances.

I also visited the Krousar Thmey, the school for blind and deaf children. The name meant New family in Khmer and it was founded in 1991 for vulnerable and orphaned children. Some of the children were blind and deaf so they created a Khmer sign language and braille. They also supported children to remain in school although they were challenged by the sudden increase in orphans during the AIDS epidemic.

When I returned to Sisophon early that afternoon I drove to the Golden Buddha Hill. It was very humid and as I puffed and sweated my way up the 358 steps, I decided I was not fit enough despite my morning runs. On the lower section of the summit was a huge gold leaf statue of Buddha, with an un-Buddha-like smile on his face, paid for by overseas Khmers.

More intriguing was a statue of a brown warrior with a helmet. His head was bowed submissively. He had a long black beard, a moustache, Khmer ears and held a gold kettle. Someone had draped a leopard skin shawl around his shoulders and looped a leopard skin shopping bag over him. I wondered if he was the God of the Sensitive New Age Guys Cambodian style and decided to ask Bo. The view of the parched plains was also spectacular, the boys herding cattle, peanuts laid out to dry, great heaps of rice straw, and tractors harvesting rice.

Driving back in the evening traffic I was vulnerable on the motorbike, like the Khmers. A big articulated truck overtook me, the back swaying alarmingly close. Then I almost ran down a pony cart and had to swerve for a street seller wheeling their cart. Three-wheeler tractors, about the speed of bicycles were towing trailers full of people. Anyone could and would stop at any time, without warning. And we all had to avoid the potholes, apart from the huge trucks that created them.

When Bo arrived, I asked him about the warrior. He was a divine being, a teacher of monks. The bag was for books, the kettle for water. Like the monks he ate just once a day. I remembered the other pilgrim with the bookbag alone on the hills of Sisophon and realised he was the same God.

On the 7th of February I was in a Poipet restaurant waiting for them to bring me fried pork, the only dish they had left. It was late, 2pm, and lunch was over.

I had just met a representative from Pearl S Buck. They counselled those who were positive and sent them to the Health Centre. The Health Centre sent those who needed further care to Mongol Borei referral hospital which was becoming overwhelmed. Many people in Poipet were migrants and would return to their home district when they got ill, so home-based care teams were not necessarily the solution. The situation analysis advocated Poipet become a separate district and recommended a hospital be established.

But I had to cross the border to pick up a friend. At long last I was going to Siem Reap.

Chapter Twelve

SIEM REAP

On the 8th of February I was in Aran to pick up a friend from Australia. She got off the bus and we went through the elaborate stone gateway at the border. As the dark man in front of me enclosed hundreds of baht in his passport and pushed it towards the custom official, I wondered if she'd noticed her first exposure to corruption in this country. We passed through without incident and then ran the gauntlet of the beggars; soldiers with crutches, a boy with elephantiasis, and another with a tiny cut on his hand, all asking for money. Although she didn't comment about this, she did mention the rubbish, which I didn't notice anymore.

We caught a taxi to Sisophon, where we slept and then the next day caught another to Siem Reap. The road was terrible and with little warning we were suddenly in the city surrounded by tour buses, white people and big hotels. We went to a restaurant, decided it was too expensive, walked to the closest with Cambodians and sat down. This was a restaurant for the drivers of the tourists eating next door, and we were told to leave.

Angkor Wat is the largest religious building in the world. It is best seen at sunset from a distance, and then with its five towers it does look like the home of the Gods, Mount Meru. However, inside the great echoing stone corridors there was a sense of loss and neglect. Squeaking bats with their musty smell and urine, had stained the stone white. I tried hard to understand the half mile long bas reliefs, the churning of the ocean of milk, heaven and hell and the depiction of numerous battles. However, I had difficulty relating to the Hinduism mythology with all its Gods. It was a tomb and it felt like one.

Suryavarman II began building this temple to Vishna in 1115 and it was completed shortly after his death in 1150. The temple city complex spanned a thousand square kilometres. In 1431 it was sacked by the Chams or Thais and fell into disuse afterwards. A more recent theory suggests inhabitants left after climate change caused a major drought.

The next day we went to the Bayon. Up on the third level in the mellow slightly golden light, I looked at the enigmatic smiles on over two hundred stone faces and cried. This was the face I had dreamed of the face of Avalokiteshvara, the Buddha of compassion.

I mentally prostrated myself before that pure and compassionate face and prayed. Prayed for the country, all those suffering, all those helping and finally prayed for healing, from the inside out, as Bob had described. When I looked up, a Khmer man was looking at me suspiciously. I nodded and looked behind him at a middle-aged American woman sitting silently beside a young Khmer man. This was a pilgrimage for them too. There was such peace and healing. It was as though the evil this country had endured and would endure could be vanquished by that face.

The Bayon was built around thirty years after Angkor Wat by Jayavarman VII who ruled from 1181-1218. He was a God-King and unified the country, building over one hundred hospitals, and over one hundred resthouses. His second wife, the elder sister of his first who had died, was Rajendradevi, a renowned poet, philosopher, and scientist. Khmer women had a more respected position in those days and our next visit to Banteay Srei confirmed it.

On Sunday we rode out on the back of motorbike taxis. We were worn out. I watched a woman sitting in the sun with a newborn who looked limp. She pulled out a bottle and began feeding the child and I wondered whether the child would survive.

Banteay Srei was pink, delicate, and intimate with finely wrought carvings. I didn't understand the stories but saw the soft, full representation of young womanhood in all its glory. The women were attended by sympathetic straight browed clean young men. I thought how much better Khmer society would be if that respect and compassion between the sexes had been maintained. As a tall, cynical, young Asian woman studied the walls her face softened. Khmer society, over one thousand years ago, was well ahead of the West, when almost the only woman celebrated was the Virgin Mary. It was the only temple not built by a King but by a counsellor to a King Jayavarman V. He was a Brahmin, a priest and doctor, also of royal descent. He began building the temple in 967.

We saw Preah Kahn in the golden light of evening. It was also built by Jayavaraman VII and provided accommodation while the Bayon was being built. The forest had melded with the stone, the roots of great trees encircled arches, and crushed, and crumbled stonework. I entered a series of dark corridors and enjoyed the Garuda, the birdman who carried Vishna. Most of the heads of the statues had gone and the bodies were uninteresting; but the stillness, the decayed grandeur, the intrusion of the forest and the columns of the library were magnificent. We were exhausted. A policeman offered my friend a coke for 100 riel, one twentieth of the normal price, attempting to revive her. It worked and we got back in time to watch the sun set over Angkor Wat.

Khmers were barbecuing on small graziers on the grass slopes by the moat, while tourists climbed the hill behind. Angkor Wat glowed golden in the setting rays. I glimpsed myself in some nearby mirror and my face had changed. I was young again.

———

When I returned to Sisophon on Tuesday the 13th of February I had meetings all day. Eap was concerned I had not reported in the day before, but I reminded him I was in Siem Reap. The meeting of the AIDS Technical Working Group was the most productive I'd attended. After splitting into three groups to work on the situation analysis, we regrouped to discuss Poipet and the border. Eap and I were to attend the cross-border talks in March, while Tess would meet the Governor to discuss the need for a District AIDS Office in Poipet. She confirmed she had access to three of the six casinos. We also learnt we had UNICEF funding for the border project in Thma Puok.

My visitor and I also travelled to Mongol Borei, me on my

motorbike and she in an NGO vehicle. She was impressed by the good roads and relative cleanliness. Arlys said they now had a rubbish collection. We toured Mongol Borei hospital as I'd been invited by the new director. It was clean, and they now had 24-hour nursing. The local nurses worked half a day at their clinics and half a day at the hospital. They had had 26 AIDS patients in the previous month. The hospital charged 10 baht a day per patient which helped buy nutritious food, clothes, essential hospital equipment and drugs. Finally, I felt the clinics could feel comfortable referring patients.

It was changing. The huge weight of the epidemic was shifting from my shoulders to the team. I would continue to support them, then slip quietly away. It was also good to be back in Sisophon. In Siem Riep as tourists, we were constantly hassled by beggars and small children selling trinkets, while down at the Sisophon market I was a local.

On Monday the 19th Feb I was in Aran with my visitor before she took the bus to Bangkok. We ate at the food stalls then returned to the hotel and discussed how I Cambodian I had become. She said I blended in because I was small and dark and I agreed, but it was more than that. I'd adopted local ways with my Buddhist shrine, incense, candle, and my sister's photo. The house had no water in the kitchen and instead I washed up outside. I spent most of my recreational time having Khmer language lessons and talking with Bo. I enjoyed doing housework, cooking, and shopping in the market where I practic ed my language. She agreed but felt I should be more relaxed. She also said I would have difficulty settling back into Australian life.

The night before we left for Poipet, we had a meal with eight MSF staff. I asked a very experienced MSF nurse if she had seen many health systems worse than Cambodia. She thought for some time and finally said South Sudan. Cambodia was challenging. We were fighting the worst AIDS epidemic in Asia with the worst health system.

———

Back in Poipet after escorting my visitor across the border, I tried to see it with a visitor's eyes. Passing the line of beggars, I saw the first had a head but no face. It must have been blown away by gunshot or a mine. I had to dodge the cargo haulers pushing heavy laden carts, while small children who could barely walk, toddled up, plucked at my trousers, and pointed to their mouths. There were also children with polio. The vaccination coverage then was 45%.

In Poipet I joined Pearl S Buck representatives for village education. They were a big international NGO with Thai experience and were now at the front line in Cambodia. We went into the back streets past the tiny, raised hutches with plastic or rice bag walls, and tarpaulins covering them. A dentist at work on one of the verandas was drilling with a wheel, the patient clutching his bloodied mouth. It was yet another possible source of transmission.

We began by showing the Khmer video I'd given them about AIDS. We were in a large hut with a loud-speaker system and as the hut filled with children, men and women filing in behind them I hoped the floor wouldn't collapse. They enjoyed the film despite its sadness. Then there was a series of speeches, shy youths asked questions, and a small but effective pamphlet was distributed. When the model penis was brought out towards the end, the youths practiced putting condoms on it.

There was a festive like atmosphere. Despite the challenge of the magnitude of the epidemic and the poor health system, we were succeeding,

On the way back to Sisophon, in a pickup, I was squashed beside a man who had been a Buddhist monk. We discussed our faiths. Cambodians were not supposed to kill, steal, lie, take drugs or alcohol, or have sex outside marriage. I was surprised. There was an AIDS epidemic because many of the men broke at least the last two rules, and Malai, the former Khmer Rouge district I was about to visit, would be no exception.

Map. This shows where we were working

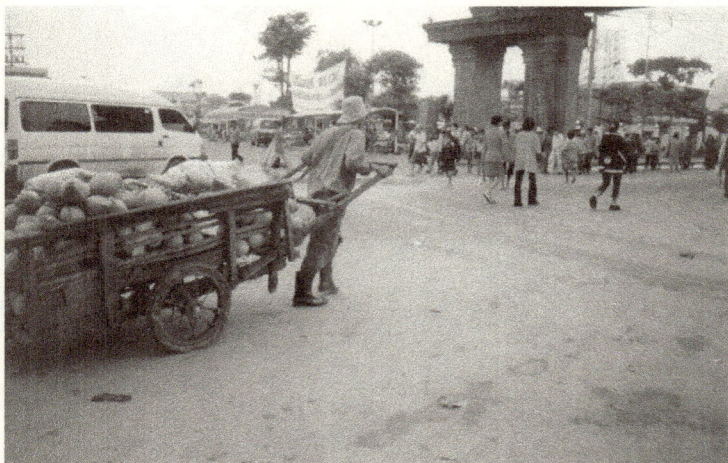

A cargo hauler in Poipet. All cargo had to be unloaded from trucks on the Cambodian side of the border, hauled by carts across the border where it was reloaded onto Thai trucks.

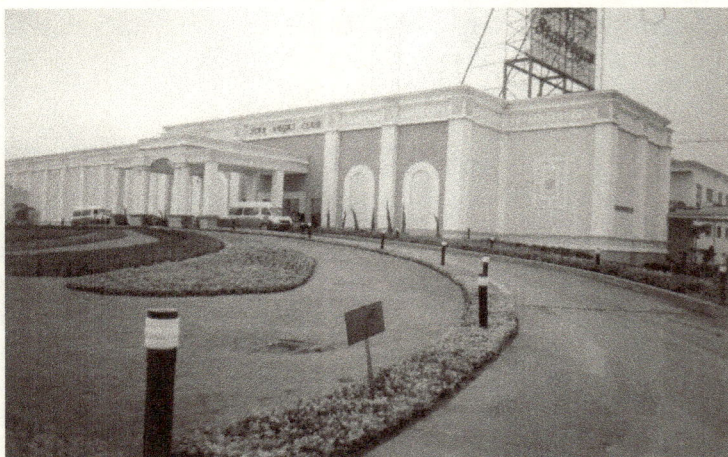

One of the six casinos in Poipet in 2000 catering only for Thais who had to cross the border to gamble. There were sex workers, illegal drugs and money laundering in these casinos which were staffed by Cambodians.

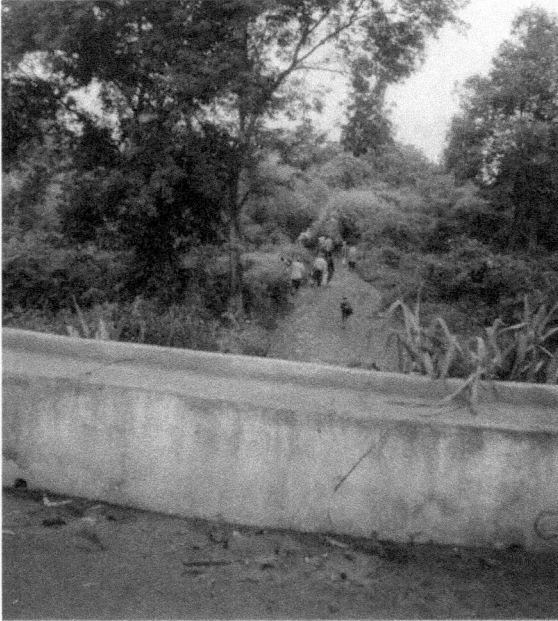

Illegal migrants from Cambodia crossing into Thailand.
Those who worked in Thailand had a hjigher incidence of
HIV than those who worked in Cambodia.

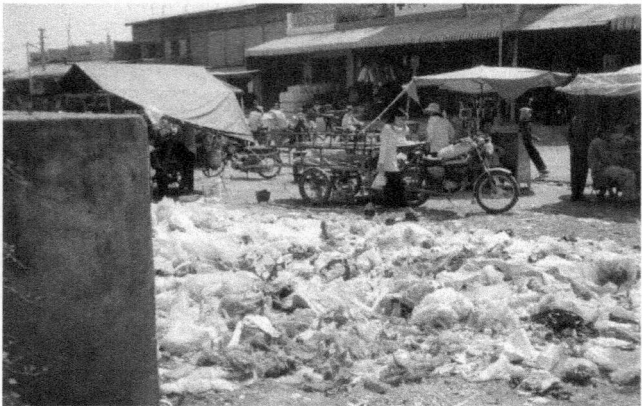

A typical market scene in Sisophon where I lived.

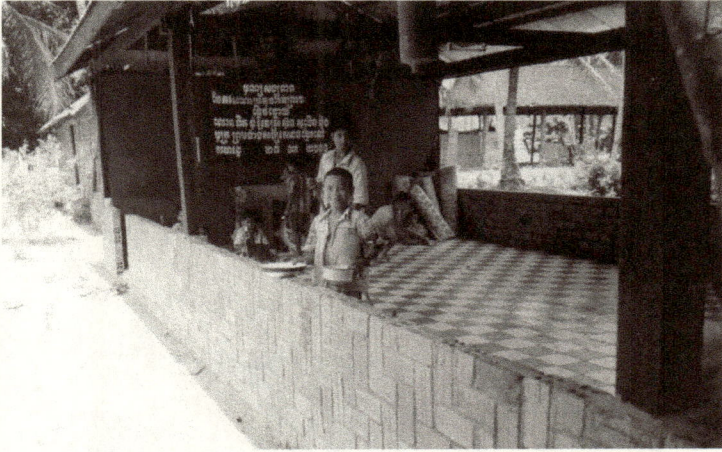

Buddhist monks cared for 40 orphans in a monastery in Battambang. Boys became monks while girls learnt to sew and had to leave when they were 12.

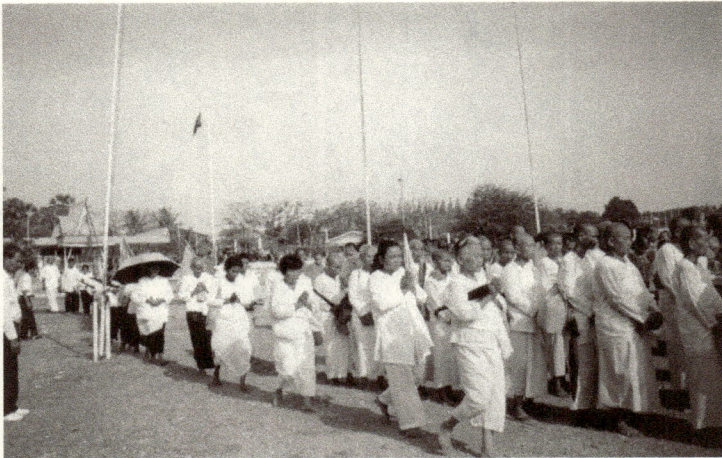

These are Buddhist elders in white robes, with monks behind them. Ninety percent of the monks in Cambodia were massacred in Pol Pot's regime in the early seventies and they were still re-establishing themselves.

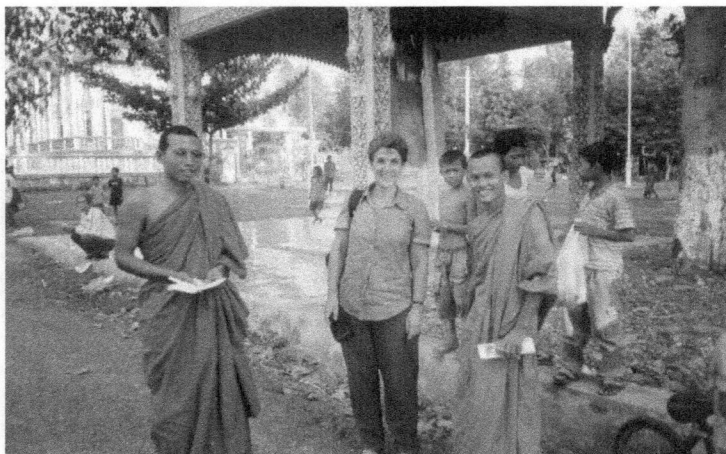

A new temple in the Battambang district paid for by overseas Khmers. Many local monks also participated in a national annual peace march and in 2000 the theme was HIV education.

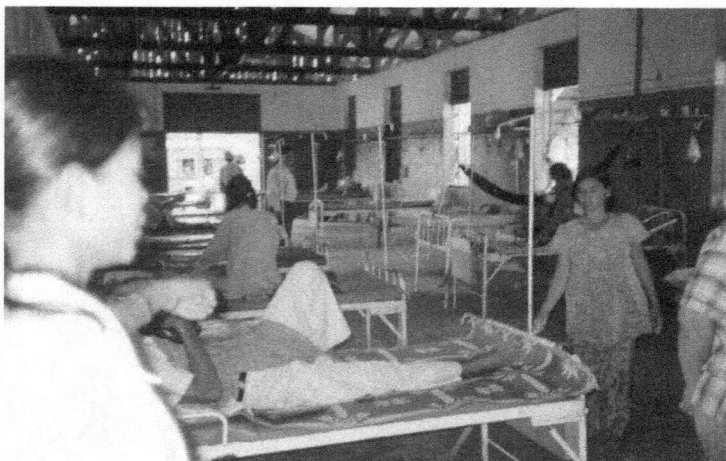

This was the hospital at Thma Puok, supported while I was there by MSF. There were an estimated 8000 people living with AIDS and a total of 8,500 hospital beds. In 2000 in Cambodia anti-retroviral medication was very expensive. There were also a lot of fake drugs.

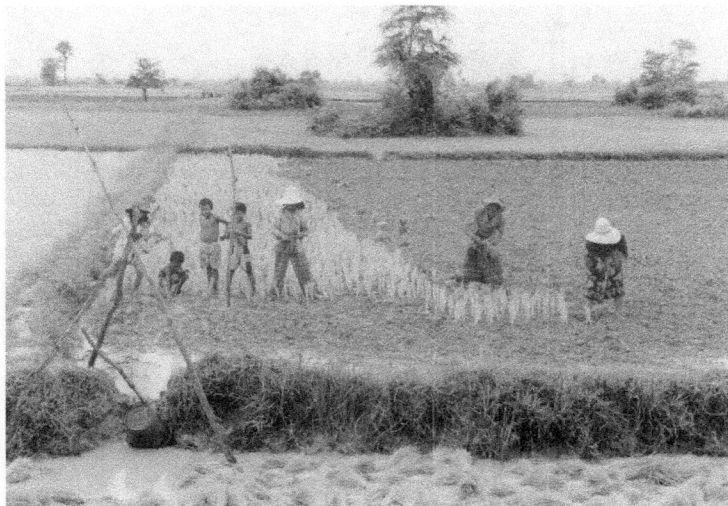

Transplanting rice seedlings at the beginning of the wet. In Cambodia they had only one rice crop per year, compared with two in Vietnam. Many of the rice fields had been demined by villagers with kitchen knives.

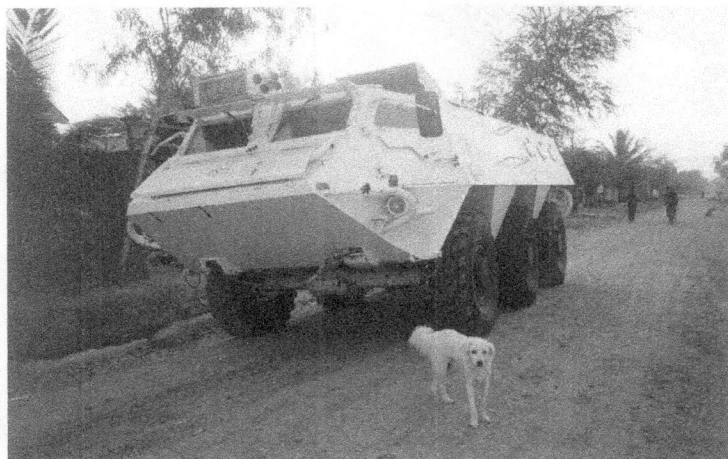

A Norwegian minesweeper in Sisophon. There were 1000 injuries from mines annually including deaths.

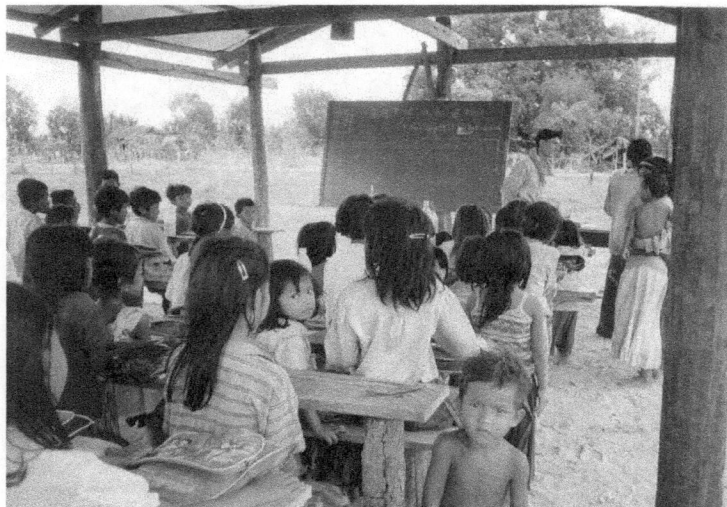

A village school sponsored by a local NGO. Only 50% of the poorest children attended primary school.

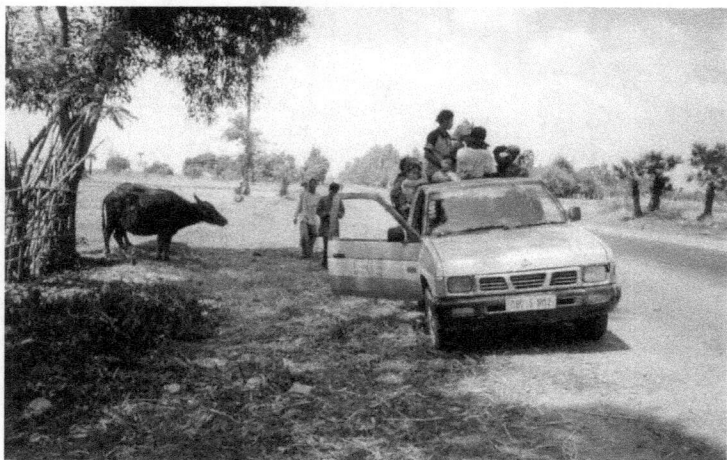

A ute, the way I travelled throughout Cambodia. I paid for a seat in the cab. If I was feeling wealthy I paid for two spaces ensuring there was just the driver and myself.

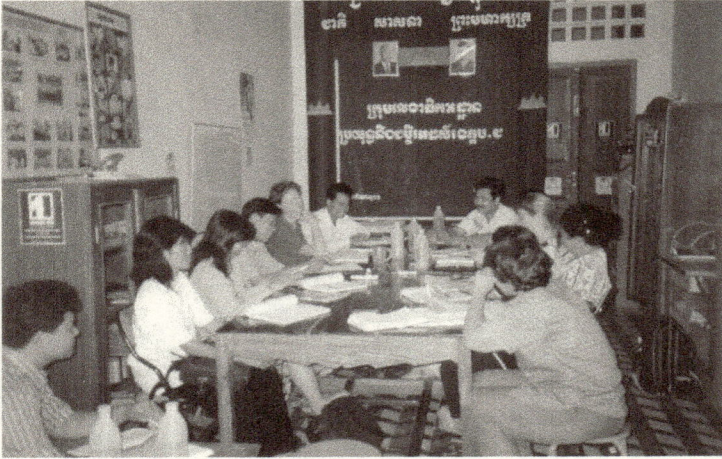

Our technical working group with Sin Eap the Director of the Provincial AIDS Secretariat chairing it alongside a doctor. Around the table are representatives from International and local NGOs.

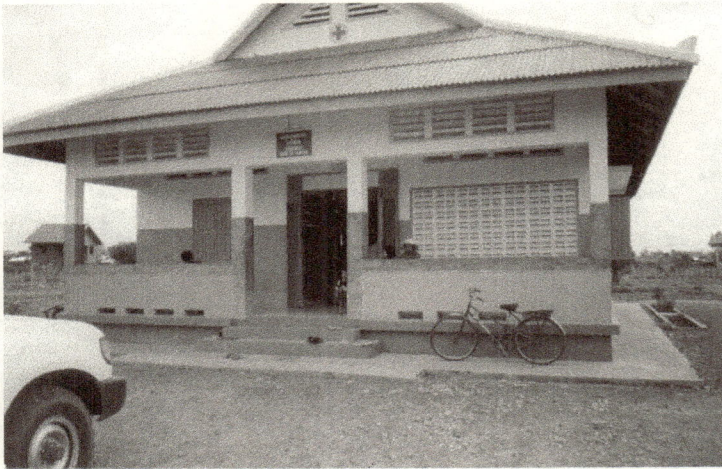

This is a newly built Area Health Centre near the Thai border. Like most rural health centres it was rarely open as the nurses were paid $US20 a month and had to find private work to survive.

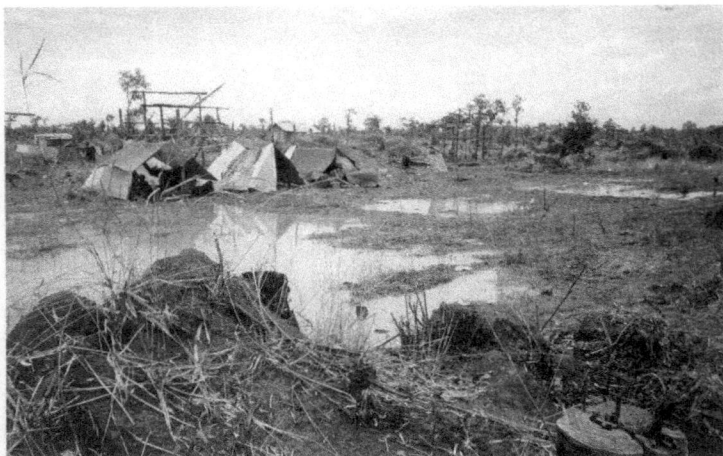

These are the tents erected by Poipet squatters after they were relocated by the military to land further out which had not been demined, and which had no water source. Most were cargo haulers and were no longer able to work. An international NGO ZOA was supporting them.

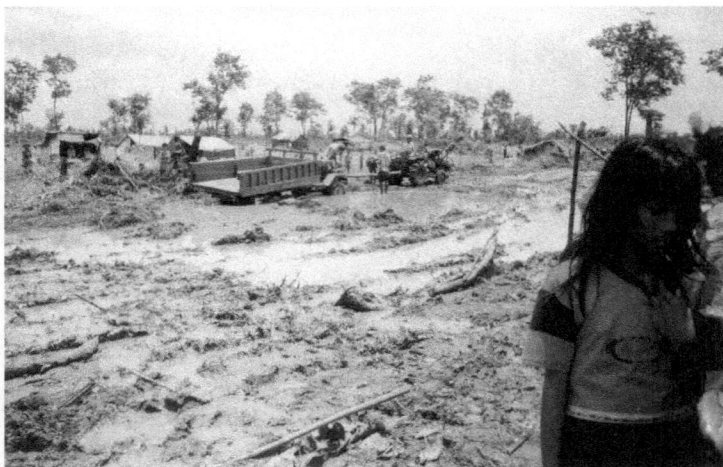

Another photo of the same site, showing a bogged truck.

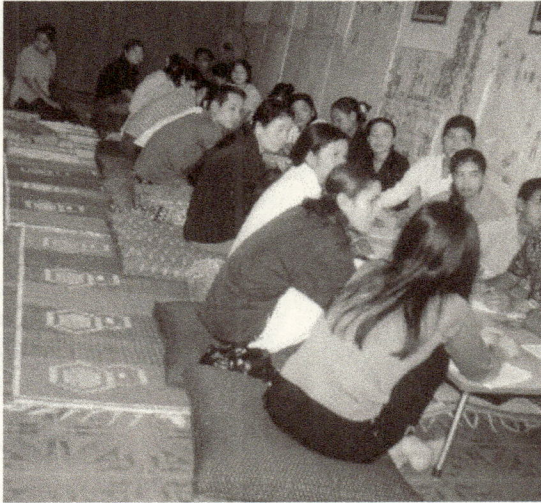

Sex workers in a Thai language class held by MSF. This allowed them to negotiate condom use more successfully with their Thai clients. Many of these sex workers were trafficked, sold by families to pay off health debts.

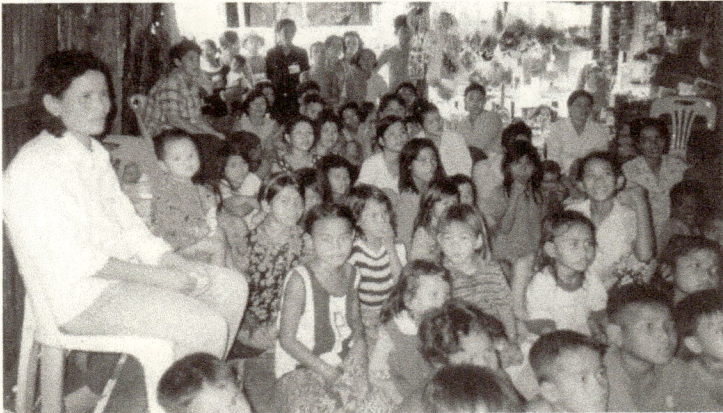

A video parlour in Poipet showing a popular video about a story of soldier returning with HIV to his family.

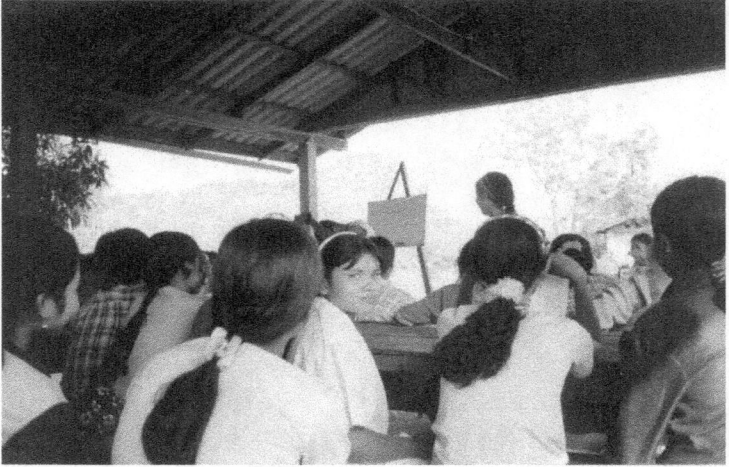

This is Sarin's niece Sopheak who after training in Phnom Penh worked with me, particularly with youths.

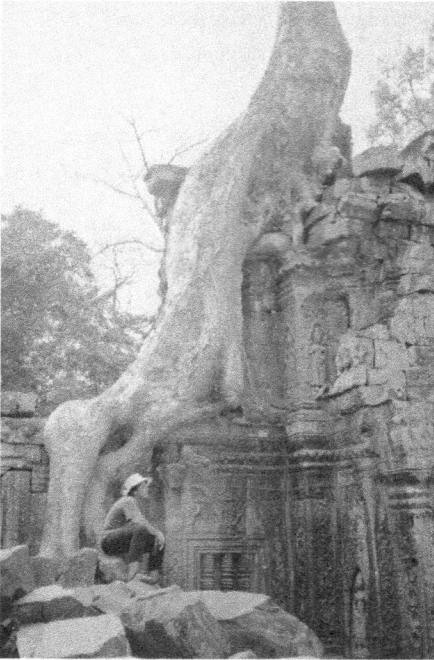

I finally got to Siem Reap, managed to escape the tourists and enjoyed communing with the ruins and nature.

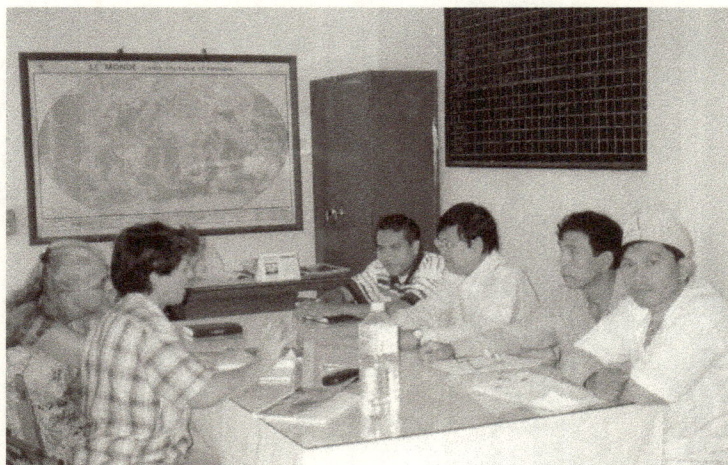

Arlys, the Director of a local NGO and myself speaking with the Director of the first home care based program in Banteay Meanchey and doctors from the local referral hospital.

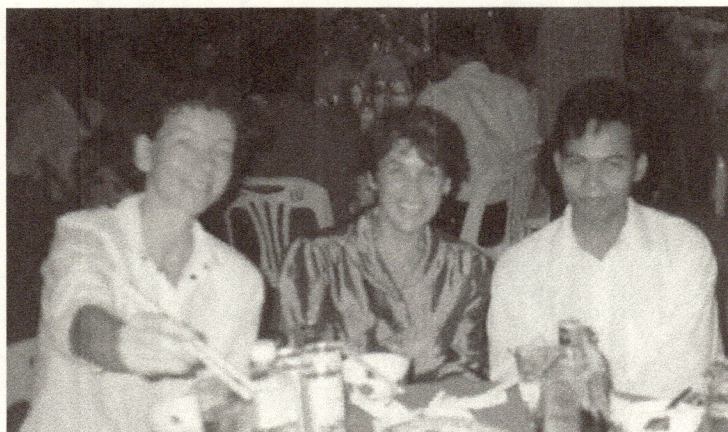

The Director of MSF, Banteay Meanchey, myself and Sin Eap having a meal together before I left.

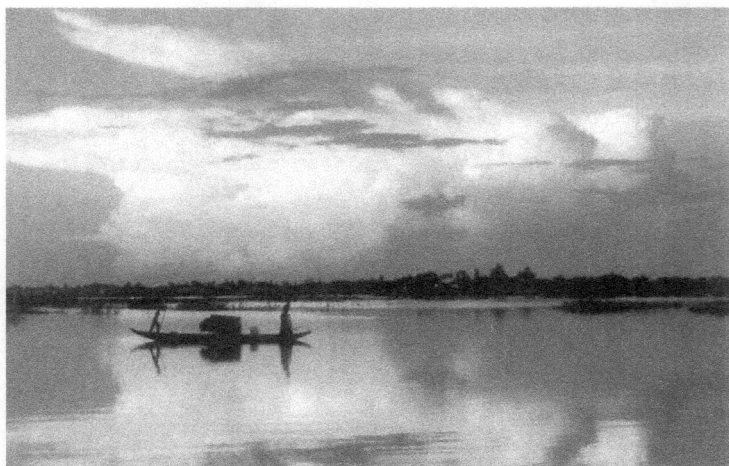

The beauty of the Mekong. I travelled down the Mekong just before I left.

Chapter Thirteen

MALAI AND KHMER ROUGE
– MARCH 2001

Malai, like Pailin, was one of the most heavily mined areas on earth. Both were former Khmer Rouge strongholds. When I'd visited Pailin World Education was working with school children with mine awareness and wanted to include HIV/AIDS awareness. They had invited me to Malai, 74 Km from Sisophon and 55 km from the Thai border. Sarin had worked in Malai as a midwife and said people were very suspicious. There was little food because there was little safe land to grow it on, so people and cows ate corn. Forewarned I brought noodles, cans of fish, a small stove, antibiotics, and malaria medication.

On 21st of February I went down the market and caught a pickup. The road was rough and there were four of us in the back including two women with babies. One baby caught the sun and looked hot, so I gave the mother my lavalava to hang over the window and my hat to shield the baby. She promptly put the hat on. The other larger baby sucked at and consumed two bananas. By the roadside they were selling small frogs and the small boy in the front seat popped one into his mouth, headfirst. I stuck to peanuts, dried pumpkin seeds and bananas.

The district was poor and there were many thatched huts, and some shanties with plastic sheeting for roofs and cardboard walls. I got out at the market and walked up a dusty road between the low wooden houses. Oxen roamed the street alone without herders. Perhaps no one dared steal them. I headed towards a flagpole in front of a yellow block building that I guessed was the school. Curious children spilled out to watch the barang or white woman, and the female food vendors stared at me from under their umbrellas.

Someone fetched the teacher and I explained who I was. He was a thin grey bookish man and like the others, surprised at my appearance. He escorted me into the dusty, high roofed classroom and as I went to sit down, hastily dusted the seat. I looked curiously at the diagrams of tapeworms and the human gut. There were charts in Khmer, a picture of Buddha and of course, the King and Queen. On another wall was the phrase, 'Hope is a choice.' When I looked down, I found he had placed two fried bananas and two fried bean curd cakes in front of me. As I ate small children came and stared at me curiously. I would have liked to go to the toilet after the rugged taxi ride but decided that was too difficult. I tried to ring World Education but there was no service so a child on a bicycle was despatched to find a motor bike taxi driver.

I ended up at an NGO office for human rights. They, alongside the Red Cross who helped trace missing persons, were the only two NGOs in town. It was very hot, and I sweated copiously as I listened to the low roll of dry thunder. I got to the toilet which connected with brick holes to the kitchen. My hostess said she was too frightened to demine the land, so she only owned the land her house was on. Others were more desperate, and many people had died or lost their limbs.

Men went to brothels in neighbouring towns and districts including Sisophon, Poipet and Sampov Loun, an hour's drive away on the Thai border. The military and police were involved in sexual trafficking and earned up to $US8000 per girl. Three young girls had recently been sold to brothels in Thailand. One was beaten by the brothel owner for not having sex with the customers, escaped, and was sent back by the Thai Police to her mother in Malai. The police and military also sold yama, an amphetamine, and domestic violence increased as it became more available.

I hired a motorbike taxi to take me to the district chiefs, and the driver asked if I had a husband, so I told him I did. He had two wives, one in Malai and another with two children in a neighbouring district. He had lost one leg below the knee when he was six and had a lower leg prosthesis with a pink plastic calf and a khaki shoe painted on. There were four labourers tearing around on motorbikes who looked at me intently and I suspected they'd been told all European women had voracious sexual appetites. I took the opportunity to give them a sheet about HIV/AIDS prevention. The district chiefs weren't at home, so I left messages with their wives.

I talked with the teachers at the Secondary School, one of whom had a beautiful young wife. He came to me for condoms afterwards. The school finished at Grade 9 and children had to complete the last three grades in Sisophon. Some parents couldn't afford to send them.

The next day I met the World Education Officers and found I'd arrived a day early. We visited a school. It was a good session, one of the best I'd attended in Cambodia. There was lots of participation and laughter as they taught the teachers how to teach children about mines. The trainers went everywhere and during the rainy season when the roads were blocked, had taken a boat to a very poor village. The children were naked and there was no school, so they held lessons under some trees. The workshop ran for two days, and they stayed for three, but had nothing to eat. The area was still forested, because of the landmines and the difficult access.

The district chiefs and I travelled to a border post on Thursday 22nd February opposite the Sa Kaeo province in Thailand. The land had been demined and the farmers had access to Thailand, so they had prospered and had big tractors and TVs. The border lay along a small river, and for less than US$1, Cambodians could cross into the nearby Thai village, but not leave Sa Kaeo Province.

The town had a settled air. People tended their gardens, orchards, and trees. I liked the relationship between men and women and felt a connection with the women who were independent and courageous. On the way out I was alone in the front seat, while everyone else jammed in the back. At lunch time we ate a lot and enjoyed ourselves, and on the way back a District Chief and an Education Chief joined me in front. The population of Malai grew during the dry season when labourers from other provinces arrived to build houses. They returned to their districts in the rainy season to plant, grow and harvest their rice. We discussed how this was another way the virus could spread.

I toured the Malai Hospital on Friday morning. They'd had

100 patients during the previous month, with mine injuries, TB, and malaria the major problems. The previous year the Director had admitted 32 people with mine injuries. There were also 15 soldiers with AIDS symptoms and seven had died. Some had been infected in Sisophon brothels. Seven people had also died after over-dosing on yama. The Hospital Director wanted more condoms and an education program. There were many questions about AIDS.

I hired a motorbike and we drove out on a convoy to visit Sampov Loun. The road was good, and we passed wooden houses, dry rice plains with a few shrubs and tree skeletons and odd shaped hills behind them. On the way we saw a flock of beautiful parrots with green plumage and red beaks.

The border village had the rawness of the frontier with snooker parlours and brothels. People crossed the border legally and illegally, while 100 daily labourers worked in Thailand. There was a smart new hospital, the Malai Santeheap Referral Hospital. One of the director's daughters worked with Catholic Relief Services (CRS) who were based there, and trained village health volunteers. A senior staff member told me there wasn't a problem with AIDS, but they had 30 to 40 cases of STIs referred monthly, mainly soldiers and their wives. This was later refuted by a medic who said there had been AIDS deaths. At the market I met a police educator. He agreed domestic violence was increasing because of the increasing use of yama, and alcohol. It could also be triggered if women complained about their husband's visits to brothels.

Sampov Loun was featured in the national media every two or three years with stories about sexual trafficking. In 2008 police rescued 16 women, three under 15, from a Sampov Loun brothel. They had been tortured by the brothel owner's sons when they refused to have sex. Anti-trafficking laws were passed in June 2008 and the police vigorously enforced them.

Malai women kept the brothels away from the Malai township. In 1997 one of the former female Commanders and her supporters, chased away the inhabitants of a Dancing Restaurant close to town. They were armed with AK47s and machetes and as the husband of the female Commander, also a Commander observed soberly, knew how to use them.

On the way back to Sisophon on Saturday in a pickup, a few trees were etched against the yellow light. It was dusty and bare and yet there was beauty everywhere including the white tips of the grass. There were thatched huts, some with clay kilns out the back. It was a productive visit and I enjoyed it.

I returned to Malai again before I left, at the invitation of a General. I also went back after the USAID visit with NGOs to visit the border areas. This was so they could prepare proposals for consideration with KHANA, the organisation which supported local NGOS to carry out community HIV prevention and care projects.

By the middle of 2022 the demining organisation CMAC declared the Malai District safe. The former minefields now had plantations, of rice, coconuts, mangoes, tamarinds, rambutan, cashews and cassavas. People flocked to buy plots of land because of the district's safety and access to Thailand. The fifty thousand people who lived in the district in 2022 were now more affluent.

Back in Sisophon that afternoon I had a craving for a fruit tukalok, a Cambodian smoothie and went to the market. Two people sat down at the next table. A pile of six duck eggs were placed in front of them. They carefully prepared a sauce of pepper sauce, lemon, and curry leaves. Then cracking the tops off the eggs, they ate them-foetuses, feathers, and all.

In the evening, I had discussion with Bo about the pros and cons of having more than one wife. Wealthy Khmer men tended to have two or three. He was glad he was poor and had just one wife; wives tended to fight, and the husband had to take care to give each one the same amount of money. The topic arose because one of the expatriates was engaged to a Khmer woman. Bo asked if he already had a European wife. I explained it was unlawful in European countries to have more than one wife. Bo told me one of his neighbours, a seventy-year-old man had recently married his third wife, a seventeen-year-old girl.

I had a lively meal on Sunday with the MSF Project Coordinator who had been to Bangkok with Eap. He hadn't travelled before and was amazed at the traffic, the escalators, the sky-train, and the effrontery of the sex workers. Bangkok was full of sex tourists, and they were told a story about a Thai sex worker who had two words of English, 'honey' and 'hungry'. She had a client and was very hungry but kept using the word honey. Finally, she pointed to her mouth, but that too could have been misinterpreted.

Eap was very excited about the Bangkok visit when I met him on Monday. He wanted the Thai sex workers' union EMPOWER, to visit Khmer sex workers to increase their confidence and negotiating skills. We also discussed the joint presentation we'd been asked to give together at an Asian-Pacific HIV/AIDS conference later that year in Melbourne. It was a fitting end to our work together.

After our meeting I walked to the lagoon I had visited after my son's friend's death. Life had returned. As I approached a herd of 20 to 30 goats, including kids, was driven by their two herders down to drink. A man washed his bicycle, while another, with long black hair like an Old Testament prophet, strode in. Women watered lettuces and spring onions, while a small girl came skipping down the path. Two ponies, released from their carts, grazed. Swallows skimmed across the water and dipped down to drink. I walked back in the gathering dark to lots of housework. This included trying to stop the rats from eating the mattress. I covered it in plastic and sprayed repellent on it.

I dreaded the PAS meeting on Wednesday because I hadn't found money for them. They surprised me by working hard and enthusiastically even though we had just $250. The PAS military representative had condoms from PSI and held awareness sessions for soldiers. Unfortunately, some of them sold the condoms to private pharmacies. We discussed giving just a few at a time.

Very early on Thursday, the first day in March, I crammed with others into the back of a pickup and left for Battambang. I fielded the question about a husband and up popped the fictitious one. After asking about my age, they stopped. Villagers were not used to single women. Women here got married at 20 and had 4 children.

I had breakfast in Battambang with a friend and then left in a taxi at 7am for Phnom Penh. I arrived exhausted and suffering culture shock. There were so many wealthy people in this city, the army officers for instance. It was just after three, and they were already in the hotels and lounging around in expensive four-wheel drives.

On Friday I was uneasy. I needed to work with KHANA to locate more local NGOS and perhaps see USAID. The US had a complex relationship with Cambodia. The US carpet bombing of the supply route to North Vietnam in the early seventies killed hundreds of thousands of people. The Americans dropped 500,000 tonnes of bombs. A million people retreated to Phnom Penh and Sihanouk, the former Prime Minister and King aligned with the Khmer Rouge. They were in power between 1975 and 1979 when the Vietnamese invaded. During that time is estimated at least 1.7 million people or one fifth of the population lost their lives.

On 14 March 1992, the United Nations Transitional Authority in Cambodia ruled for 18 months to stabilise the country so democracy could be established.

At that stage there were two major parties FUNCINPEC and the current ruling party the CPP. There were tensions between the two and in July 1997 FUNCINPEC launched a coup attempt. There was two days of fighting in Phnom Penh with dozens of FUNCINPEC officials killed and hundreds of civilians wounded. At that stage US suspended all non-humanitarian aid to Cambodia. Thirty thousand Cambodians fled to Thailand to escape the fighting. The US embassy however did not provide asylum to Cambodians facing political persecution.

Despite this the US was a critical partner as they bought Cambodia's cheap clothes. In 2000 there were 190 foreign owned garment factories in Cambodia. Garment exports accounted for 77 percent of Cambodia's total exports in 2000 and earnt $US 985 million. The garment exports continued growing until 2004 when quotas were established.

Instead of meeting the USAID officials I sat in a WHO meeting and learnt about the other health problems in Cambodia. This included the practice of feeding newborns sugar water rather than suckling them, and the fact that 52% of the children under 5 in Cambodia were malnourished compared to the South-East Asian average of 38%. I raised the issue of beri beri and the very sick baby in Thma Puok. One of the doctors replied it was not uncommon for babies to be admitted near death. They were saved by a Vit B injection. He thought more study was needed.

Back at the hotel reading the local papers, I found donor roads had been smashed by overloaded trucks, fishing rights stolen, pesticide use was increasing, and World Food Program food supplies went missing. Did anything go right?

On Monday 5th March, I finally met the USAID representatives. I was very relieved. At last, I had met an organisation with the power to change things. They were on their way to Banteay Meanchey. I had been in Cambodia almost a year and this was the best gift we could be given.

The next day I reported I was working hard and had released an avalanche of support. We've now had five organisations coming down, USAID, Asian Foundation, World Food Program, Cambodian Red Cross and FHI. I had to keep my mobile on, which I had avoided most of my life. I always preferred to work on one thing at a time.

While I was in Phnom Penh, I talked with a young volunteer who had been airlifted out of the Solomons. They found a headless body in the market and then a Guadalcanal man was pulled out of a bank and beaten severely. A regular boat took the Malaitan women and children back to Malaita and returned with men and youths. The volunteer woke up one evening hot and heard shouts. When she opened the door, she saw four houses across the narrow street were on fire. It took half an hour for the fire engines to arrive because they had to be paid. When the firemen arrived, they were directed by bystanders. I worried about George, my ex-husband, who was there. He finally managed to get a letter through to us. He had been in a very difficult situation and was helped by a South Malaitan relative.

On Saturday I had a gruelling journey back in a pick-up. I waited in a pickup for an hour at a market as more people and goods were bundled into the cab and onto the back. A Thai woman, quite tall, spent nine hours doubled up in the back seat with three other people and her suitcase. She paid for one place. After driving for three hours, the pickup slowly loosing speed, we stopped. The driver fiddled with electrical plugs under the dashboard and the cabin filled with black smelly smoke. Finally, they push-started it and we limped along until lunchtime. Then someone fixed it up.

There were numerous stops to pee along the roadside (you

needed a lavalava), a breakfast stop, a lunch stop, and a half hour wait because a bridge had broken. We were at the back of a queue of fifty to sixty trucks, with the same queue on the other side. Then we had the checkpoints. We paid to cross railway lines, paid to go down dips, paid to go over bridges, and paid at police checkpoints. Apparently, the train is slower, but I haven't got time for that.

Back in Sisophon on Sunday 11th March I was relieved to come back to a pink fresh Sunday morning; fresh because after four months, it had finally rained. In the early morning, I ran up the hill. The earth had soaked up the rain and there were patches on the road. A puppy ran alongside me. It began to spit so I returned to the market and sat on a plank. I watched the vendors setting up sheets of plastic to funnel the rain, now drumming heavily on the corrugated iron, into buckets. Some spilt over and rivulets formed, carrying the muddy water and rubbish around my feet.

When the rain stopped, I walked back and found some white flowers with an exquisite smell in my garden.

I was glad of the rain but hoped we wouldn't get bogged during the USAID visit.

Chapter Fourteen

DONORS RETURN
– MARCH TO APRIL 2001

I spent one day, the 15th March with four representatives from USAID, and knew it was the most critical day of the 18 month project. FHI organised the meeting for USAID in Poipet, and the District Governor attended. He wanted an AIDS District Committee in Poipet and said he was happy with ZOA's work. However, he also said that land in Poipet was becoming too valuable to be allocated to NGOs.

We also discussed the problems of providing home care without health staff support, and the lack of reliable HIV testing centres including the high number of false positives. MSF were concerned about the bondage of sex workers by brothel owners, and the poor performance of the government health centre in Poipet. MSF then raised their concerns around the 100 % condom program, including the lack of consent, police involvement and the problems of the presumptive approach, which did not include diagnosis and treatment of all the common STIs. The USAID representatives agreed there were human rights concerns with the program.

The USAID representatives then toured a CARE project

(Cooperative for Assistance and Relief Everywhere). CARE is an international NGO, and in Cambodia predominantly worked in garment factories in Phnom Penh. They trained peer educators and supported thousands of garment workers with information about sexual reproductive and maternal health. After staying overnight in Sisophon, they left for Battambang the next morning.

On 10th April 2001, I received a letter from the Phnom Penh Office of USAID thanking me for meeting them.

Your willingness to discuss important health issues in the Cambodian context has helped USAID Cambodia's Office of Public Health to assess its current portfolio and start to develop a new long-term strategy given the realities of the current health situation in Cambodia.

By October 2001 they had released their strategy for Cambodia for 2002 to 2005. It led to the establishment of three clinics in Banteay Meanchey and more support for KHANA.

KHANA (Khmer HIV/AIDS NGO Alliance) is an NGO which in 2003 provided support to over 40 NGOs working in the HIV/AIDS and STI field.

Two days before USAID arrived, Eap and I attended the first meeting of the Provincial 100% condom working group. Others attending included an official from the Ministry of the Interior, the Head of Police in the Province, and the Third Deputy Governor.

The 100% condom program was launched in 13 provinces including Banteay Meanchey and Battambang in 2002, but with the presumptive approach there were problems with comprehensive treatment as MSF had told USAID. The presumptive approach used in Sihanoukville had consisted of asking sex workers monthly if they had a discharge. If they did, the clinic tested for trichomoniasis and syphilis, but not chlamydia or gonorrhoea. Untreated chlamydia and gonorrhoea could lead to inflammatory pelvic disease and infertility. Presumptive treatment could be used in the short-term but was not a long-term solution.

The 100 % condom program was not effective in preventing the spread of STIs amongst sex workers, according to research carried out on over one thousand sex workers from eight provinces in 2005. Samples were taken for syphilis, chlamydia, and gonorrhoea. Although the sex workers reported 80% condom use with clients, only 38% of them used condoms with sweethearts and casual partners. The prevalence of syphilis was 2.3%, chlamydia was 14.4%, gonorrhoea 13% and STIs in general 24%. The results were lower than in 1996, but the same as a similar study in 2001.

———

On the 18th of March I went to see Sarin. I was concerned she didn't yet have an obstetrician and she said she would find one in Mongol Borei. She had a taxi driver nearby who could take her. Her husband asked Sopheak and I to provide education to the orphanage staff, so we scheduled it for the following week. Sopheak came to lunch, and we went through the material.

I then left to see the Enfants de Mekong about an orphaned

infant Bo has spoken about the night before. She was a one-year-old from Pailin. Her parents had died from malaria, and their four children would be split up. Bo said he and his wife didn't have the resources or ability to care for her because they already had four children. Enfants de Mekong looked a reasonable place, but they said they couldn't take her until she was two and walking well.

Walking onto the orphanage I gave the children, all 46 of them, a pack of nibbles. Some of the girls wanted to go for a walk so we climbed a hill. On top they gathered edible leaves, and we found some of the boys shuffling around with a broken football. I bought two new balls. A young volunteer football coach trained them three afternoons a week.

That evening Bo told me the grandfather and mother of the small girl would take her, while their other three children, all young adults over 20, would look for work in Thailand.

On Friday the 23rd I had permission to borrow the WHO Director's driver and vehicle. We drove to Tuol Pongro in Malai and I took a representative from the CWCC (Cambodian Womens Crisis Centre). They worked at border crossings to monitor and support women and children encountering trafficking and violence and were considering working there. A couple of weeks earlier, I had contacted Cambodian Family Development Services, an international NGO based at Tuol Pongro. They supported income generation, food security and provided counselling. They were happy to meet with CWCC representatives.

On the way we passed a school without walls and stopped. There were 96 children and two volunteer teachers. There was a teacher but as he had to make money, he worked in Thailand every day and could only teach after 4pm.

While there, we heard a couple of soldiers had been shot the previous month. My language teacher said rival Khmer Rouge factions were still fighting. Malaria remained a major concern, and at one health centre the nurses said they were unable to get bed nets.

On Saturday afternoon, 24th March I was relaxing in a small snooker parlour, drinking coconut, eating dried bananas, and watching children play in the heavy rain. It was five and growing dark. All morning I'd been working on the situation analysis with Arlys, Eap, and an NGO representative from CHRD (Cambodian Human Resource Development). Youth and counselling programs were a major gap. We had no donor and no expertise in this area. Later I met a social anthropologist Graham Forde, and he subsequently published a comprehensive survey of youth in Cambodia.

◊———

Sarin invited me to the Chinese Tomb sweeping day a week early on the 25th of March. The family would visit her Chinese husband's parent's graves at Mongol Borei near the family home where his sister lived. Sarin said she could go into labour at any time and once she'd given birth, she and the baby had to stay at home for a month.

Sopheak, her sister, the men, children, and I travelled on the back of a truck with a sucking pig. A heavily pregnant Sarin and her daughter got into the passenger seat, and four ladies and their babies squashed into the back of the cab.

Sopheak explained why she hadn't been able to work yesterday. She looked like she had impetigo around her eye, but they were small fluid filled burn blisters. While striking a match, a burning fragment hit her above the eye.

We arrived at the semicircular concrete graves and unpacked the sucking pig, a chicken, rice, apples, grapes and oranges, and dainty goblets for beer and Chinese tea. Incense and candles were lit, and we prayed at the graves and shared the food with the dead. We also burnt lucky money and papers representing clothes. When we arrived at the sister in law's house with the remnants of the food, Sarin told me she had an obstetrician.

It rained heavily as we returned in the tray of the pickup, the rain like flints flying into our faces. The sky was full of thunderous clouds, the light was yellow, the ploughed fields sodden, and the muddy canals flowing fast. When I got back to the house I changed and slept. It was still raining.

———·———

On Monday morning I was at CARERE with a skinned elbow. I had made an ambitious attempt on my motor bike to mount a concrete ledge and was sent sprawling into the mud. I picked myself up and smiled sweetly at the men staring at me from the back of a pickup. At least they didn't run me over.

A pretty consultant staying in one of the cheaper hotels had at least five different people battering at her door overnight. At 3am she shouted, 'Go away or I'll kill you.' They must have understood English or perhaps it was her tone. She was left in peace.

I was woken at 4.30am by two one hundred-day commemorations, one on either side. There were tinkling wat bells on one side and on the other wailing monks. This was a common celebration in Cambodia as it took one hundred days for the soul of the deceased to be ready for their next rebirth.

It was a fitting start for National Culture Day. The streets were blocked off, there were soldiers everywhere and the Ministries were closed. The female consultant couldn't do anything. The WHO Doctor knew about it and was still in Aran.

That evening, I asked my language teacher about the day, and we discussed the preservation of Khmer culture. Much of it had occurred in monasteries. Many of their manuscripts were burnt and thrown into the Tonle Sap during Pol Pot's time. The few monks who survived scratched what they knew on bark and leaves and the Ministry of Culture had begun to assemble it. Overseas Khmer were also sending back material. There were Khmer Schools of culture in the US supported by US Universities.

By Wednesday afternoon I had vomiting and diarrhoea, giardia again. The sky was orange, the wind getting up and tossing the palm leaves. I was sick but my brain never stopped. We were still working on the situation analysis, and Eap and I had to get a presentation together for Melbourne. I had a soft drink, then vomited. Good. Perhaps that would stop me buying them. They were expensive, unhealthy, and unnecessary.

A week later, the 4th of April. UNICEF officially agreed to support the pilot project for Thma Puok. I went up on the 9th April and spoke with the Director of the AIDS program. He was working with the health centres and their services were improving. In Boeung Trakoun the Health Centre was providing STI treatment for both sex workers and housewives, and in one Health Centre a Health Centre Chief was giving counselling to confirmed HIV positive cases. The MSF Doctor told me the number of AIDS cases they were treating for opportunistic infections had doubled from 80 last year to 160.

Suddenly I found myself attending a wedding with the groom from the States and a local girl with MSF. She was heavily made up and there were many changes of costume. We had a table near the back, the Director of the AIDS program looked after me, and it was hot and muggy. The MSF doctor was leaving next week, and I would miss her.

On the 13th April Good Friday, I had lunch with Edith and then went to see Sarin. She had given birth the day before to a little red skinned boy with a shock of black hair and was in a stuffy, small room. I was surprised to find her bottle feeding, but it was sugar water, the cultural practice the WHO doctors had discussed. Medical science favoured breast feeding as the first milk, the colostrum, contained antibodies and vital nutrients. However, the baby slept all night and all day, either because of the sugar water or the heat.

Sarin was only allowed rice porridge with strong herbs including ginger and would remain on the diet for two to three weeks. She was concerned the ginger would taint her breast milk. She and the baby had to be hot, and I learnt later this was called roasting. She had a blanket after delivery and was wearing a cardigan although it was the hottest time of year. She was not allowed to bath for 7 days, comb her hair, or clean her teeth.

They wanted to light a fire under her bed, but she refused. She thought she and the baby already had heat stress and she wasn't allowed a fan. She couldn't afford disposable nappies and so she was using muslin which was not very absorbent. The baby had cotton boxing gloves to stop him scratching his face. After I'd commiserated with her, she told me it served her right for marrying a Chinese.

Roasting was a Khmer custom, the theory being it was necessary to restore the warmth which was lost in delivery and to 'cook the body's strings.' These were the muscles and ligaments that had worked hard and grown 'cold' during childbirth. Roasting for three days to a month improved overall health after birth and abortions. A survey of 15,000 women in 2000 stated that almost 90% of Khmer women practised roasting for at least three days after birth, including over sixty percent of educated women.

That evening, I attended a party for the baby, ate a lot of cake and enjoyed myself. I was warned not to walk to isolated places over Khmer New Year and to be careful of motorbike taxi drivers. People were looking for money. A teacher in Poipet had been robbed and killed.

Later the WHO Doctor also told me about a fire opposite his house. Twenty-four houses had been burnt and 4 people were dead, one Indian and three Khmers. They couldn't unlock their doors to escape and there was looting. Bo told me his eldest brother's house had been burnt in this fire. He was a mechanic. Apparently, it was deliberately started after a love affair went wrong, and the police had made an arrest.

I noticed one of the doctors lunching with soldiers and later met with the PSI representative. Under the WHO program PSI had given large numbers of condoms to the senior military who then sold them on the private market. In Banteay Meanchey they would follow the protocol they used in Siem Reap, and give individual soldiers condoms, a few at a time.

I also met the COERR representative. (Catholic Office for Emergency Relief and Refugees). In Banteay Meanchey they supported the elderly and youths. The Director considered hiring Sopheak as a translator for their vocational centre for youths which catered for up to one hundred. At the same time, she could provide an HIV/AIDS awareness program.

On Saturday the 7th I was back in Thma Puok. The MSF doctor was flying back to Holland late the following week. She would be sorely missed. We had a farewell party. Edith ate lots of Dutch marshmallows while I produced a good bottle of Australian wine.

While I was in Thma Puok I went to see the soldiers with the military representative from the Provincial PAS. I said I was more relaxed than I had been a few months earlier. I had convinced myself I could do the job. He said he felt the same. He was surprised people had confidence in him, but they did. We also discussed the condom supplies from PSI and their advice they be distributed a few at a time. He worked despite getting no payment. We went to see a military man and sat together under a tree with his wife, daughter while his mother peeled vegetables.

Walking down a dusty street I noticed they were digging big drains on either side ready for the wet. I was relaxed and happy and enjoyed the white cumulus clouds piled high in the sky. Soon it would be Easter, soon it would be Khmer New Year.

On Monday 9th April I was at a meeting of the Provincial Health Staff from the North-West Region. There were representatives from provinces ranging from Pursat to Oddar Meanchey with a team from the Planning Unit in Phnom Penh. They told us financial management had improved and was now measured against outcomes. There was a need for a mix of effective public and private services. The public system could get worse if funding didn't improve. Health Centres with feedback committees functioned more effectively, while user paid health centres could offer more services.

I talked with the Director of Health, Pailin. They had an NGO arriving, funds for the Provincial AIDS Secretariate and were starting a 100% condom program.

 On Monday I reflected on the sun and moon as I ran up the hill in the early morning. As the red sun rose, the clouds sailed across the full moon. There was a need for both day and night, both action and repose. My life was all action.

Tuesday 10th April was my last working day before Khmer New Year and Easter, and the second day of the Northwest Regional Meeting. The participants were out in the field and would report back in the afternoon. It was sad to hear patients from Oddar Meanchey Hospital sometimes died while they were transported to referral hospitals in Thailand, Battambang and Mongol Borei. As in Pailin, they had resistant strains of malaria.

I went to see Sopheak and passed an old man who was angry and clutching his half-eaten sugar cane. Three small boys had been hurling small hard fruit at him, which lay scattered around his feet. In pidgin Khmer I admonished them, "Not good, not good." They retired giggling, probably at my awful Khmer, and the old man assumed a righteous look.

Back at my house on my veranda I looked over my gate at a pony. They were often tethered there eating the grass on the verge. The bells around its neck tinkled as it grazed. Insects, flies perhaps, were troubling it, and it kept flicking its head.

I was looking forward to Khmer New Year and my trip to Thailand.

Chapter Fifteen

TURNING THE TIDE, OVERLOOKED
BORDER TROOPS – MAY 2001

I was woken early by a noisy rooster outside. It was the second morning of my holiday, and I was in Trat, Thailand, three and a half hours drive south of Aran. It was a small room in a cheap hostel, and I'd heard every rustle, and every cough of my neighbours on either side. Instead of taking the ferry to Ko Chang the day before I'd stayed to get a haircut.

I was exhausted, tired of new impressions, constant interactions, endless learning, and problem solving. I wanted to stop and reflect. Instead, I took the ferry to Ko Chang packed with backpackers and Thais with radio and came straight back. I found the resorts, buses, and ferries full of young westerners consumed by their petty concerns irritating. It worried me. I wondered how I would fit back into Australia.

There was an exception though, a conversation I overheard between an Englishman and his son. He'd just been accepted for Oxford and this holiday was his reward. The older man spoke of the strategy MSF used to get their staff, held hostage, out of Chechnya. Then he talked about pluralism. He told his son it was about encouraging people at all levels in society, to have input into decisions which affected them.

That was what we were doing. We were supporting districts, communes, and villages to look at their own problems and develop their own solutions. It was difficult in Cambodia with the distrust remaining from Pol Pot's time. But in an emergency, it was the only way to effectively mobilise a society. It also strengthened civil society when a AIDS epidemic threatened to tear it apart. As a catalyst I learnt to trust the process. Often, I'd gone into a situation not knowing what I could do. In that moment between me and the other, a solution materialised. One of my colleagues called it white space. I believed it was the same openness to the higher power which called me over.

After a couple of days rest in Aran I was back in Sisophon, on Easter Sunday April 15th. I woke after another vivid dream. My sister Sue was alive again and my father was with her. We were building a new house for her. She was gentle and strong. Her presence was often with me in Cambodia.

———·—

Back at work the next week we had meetings with a UNICEF consultant who was setting up District Child Protection Committees. Arlys knew of 150 orphans in the Mongol Borei District, just one of seven districts in Banteay Meanchey Province. It was estimated there were 55,000 nationwide.

In my discussions with Bo, I kept hearing about broken families and vulnerable children. In mid-April, he told me about a 35-year-old Khmer woman who had arrived in Sisophon from a border province near Vietnam. She was married but her husband took another wife and moved to Sisophon. She left their three-year old with her parents and came to look for her husband. When she found she had lost him, she sold their infant son for $US25 to a family with infertility problems. She then went to Thailand as a builder's labourer. He told me one of the recent funerals was for a 24-year-old woman who got very angry when her husband gambled at cards, lost their money and her wedding ring. She died by suicide leaving him alone with their two small children.

My language tutor said in these complex family situations children were sometimes overlooked. Sometimes a family member supported them and sometimes they ran away and became street children.

Bo was helpful in practical ways too. Once while we were talking, he noticed a large scorpion with its tail raised running towards the front door and killed it with a broom handle.

The UNICEF consultant who rented my top floor, also told me about the hotels she stayed in Sihanoukville and Phnom Penh. In both there were 15 young girls who had been bought from orphanages and would be sold to the sex trade. I hope that wasn't the fate of the orphans in Sisophon. I understood why it was important to support children to remain in their communities.

Many children needed protection. The most comprehensive study of childhood abuse took place in 2013 when around 2400 adolescents (13 to 17) completed a survey and over 100 participated in qualitative research. The survey found more than half of all Cambodian children had experienced physical violence before 18, and a quarter emotional abuse. Around 5% had been sexually abused.

The protection of children was the aim of the Commune Committees formed in 2004 for women and children (CCWCs). They reported to officials in the Ministry of Social Affairs/ Veterans and Youth. A consultant from World Vision reviewed their progress in 2016. The committees supported children to stay in school, escape domestic violence, and took perpetrators to court. They also advised about unsafe migration. They had little money and their members lacked technical training, but they met monthly and did what they could.

———

While the general HIV prevalence rate decreased to 2.6% in 2002, and new HIV positive cases dropped from 40,000 in 1994 to 7000 in 2002 transmission between husbands and wives was increasing, because of 'sweethearts.' My language teacher had told me romance and marriage weren't compatible in Cambodia, so instead many married men had 'sweethearts'. Sometimes too, the wives had boyfriends. While 90% of men wore condoms with commercial sex workers in 2002, only 37% wore them with sweethearts. In 2002 the rate of transmission from husbands to wives was 42%, and the most common way HIV was spread. Nationally a third of married woman didn't believe they could refuse sex if their husbands were HIV positive. Less than 1%

of married couples used condoms because as Sopheak told me condoms were associated with brothels.

The rate of maternal to child transmission was the second highest rate of transmission at 2.8%. Transmission could be stopped with antiretroviral treatment but in 2002 there were 4,536 HIV positive pregnant women and just over 2% had access to antiretrovirals.

In Sisophon on the 25th April I went with Sopheak to one of her awareness sessions. She encouraged participation, was confident and answered audience questions well. They enjoyed themselves and practiced condom use with wooden models.

We also continued with the situation analysis and discussed the need for people to understand their basic anatomy. This included awareness sessions for primary schools as many girls didn't get a secondary education.

The Khmers were horrified. Culturally it was inappropriate to discuss sex in public. However, without age-appropriate education I felt Cambodian children, particularly girls, would be vulnerable. UNFPA made the same point in 2016. They pointed out that youth between 10 and 14 were 35% of the population, and without sexual health education they were vulnerable to STIs, pregnancy and sexual violence. Twelve percent of girls between 15 and 19 were mothers. Since 2013 UNFPA have supported the Ministry of Education Youth and Sport with the Life Skills Education Program in 25% of the upper primary and secondary schools in the country and this has now been expanded.

In late April I rode to Poipet on the back of a pickup to meet the Thai sex workers union members. MSF had invited them from Bangkok with Eap's support. The organisation was called EMPOWER, a fitting name, and that was what they'd come to do with the local sex workers.

It had rained, the air was fresh, and the dust settled. The sky looked like an old Dutch painting with sombre, towering clouds. Poipet was quiet, many people had moved, voluntarily or involuntarily, from the centre of town. There were still sex workers milling around the taxi pickup. Close by was the barber, supplied by MSF, who sold 7000 condoms a month . The MSF Director told me they had contacted most of the casual sex workers, as the Department of Health supervised brothel workers with the 100% condom program.

At the door to the nightclub, we met the night-time condom seller. The singers, in very short dresses, were stepping gently in unison military style, and waving their arms. The music was dreary and very loud while the bright white flashing strobe lights caught people suddenly in their beam, like startled deer. The male faces were grim and bored. They were circling around the young girls some of whom who looked around 12. I studied a couple nearby, a very young girl and a man who didn't know what to say to her.

Despite the grim atmosphere the five Thai sex workers enjoyed themselves. They were comfortable with their sexuality, natural and graceful. Both the MSF Director and I were delighted. One, a tall woman, long legged, bespectacled with long black hair, with an executive secretary type look, began moving her lithe, light body. A girl in the band looked jealous. Perhaps her partner was ogling her.

Then there was the woman with the pale oval face, like a fragile egg, hair pulled back and plucked eyebrows. She laughed a lot and read palms and had found her boyfriend that way. She told an anxious Khmer woman of 37 that she would have a boyfriend before she was 40.

A short, well-built, young woman was flirting with one of the male NGO workers. She had been a bonded sex worker but escaped and found EMPOWER. She had an expressive face, broken English and was disgusted by the spit under the table. In Thailand she supported sex workers when they needed to go to hospital.

As in Cambodia some of the Thai sex workers were HIV positive not because of their clients, but their boyfriends. In Thailand female condoms were 50 baht, too expensive the girls said. One of the MSF staff members had tried one with her husband and said it rustled like lettuce.

We then visited a brothel, with plywood walls and tiny cubicles, just wide enough for a single bed. The Thais checked the mattress. This brothel was for poor men, those who could not afford to marry. The young girls looked drugged, and probably were. We spoke with a transgender person, the first I'd met. They had been a cook and worked in Siem Reap. After midnight we were back in the hotel in an airless room, two female MSF staff and I. Outside women and men were laughing and a man singing. Poipet came alive at night.

The following afternoon the Thai girls gave the locals lessons, including putting on condoms with their mouths, sexy looks, lap dancing, and shrugging their shoulders so their breasts looked bigger.

The sex workers said sometimes they were unable to convince their clients to wear condoms and very little research was done on this. Finally in 2008 PSI carried out a behavioural survey called 'Let's go for a walk' It studied the sexual decision making amongst clients of female entertainment workers in Phnom Penh, using 45 men aged between 18 and 45.

Many Khmer men valued pleasure indulgent masculinity and usually the leader of the group was in this category. They indulged in heavy drinking and female conquest. They often pooled their money. This implied commitment to 'the walk,' and often they did not take condoms. Lower ranking men like labourers, planned their budget for the sexual activity and drank after rather than before.

The other model was self-restrained masculinity, where men respected women and their families. In Khmer culture at that time, this was less valued by men. The report suggested, messaging and condoms be available in commercial sex establishments and men be encouraged to have sex prior to engaging in heavy drinking.

The driver, and former health worker I had spoken with on my trip to Pailin told me that before Pol Pot few Cambodian men frequented brothels but that changed after Pol Pot. They were living in the survival mode and pleasure came first. There was also a big gender gap, although less so in the former Khmer Rouge areas. Women there had shut down some of the closer brothels and the men were forced to travel.

Back in Thma Puok on the 2nd of May I went to see the hospital. They were staggering on without a doctor. While I was there seven people died suddenly, four of them from one family, a possible poisoning. A Department of Health team had been sent to investigate. They also had a dengue outbreak.

We drove to Boeung Trakoun to meet a military Commander. He was a large man, flanked by his two much slighter medical assistants. They worked out of a large hospital with 67 staff, established while the Americans were there. He had 2000 troops, some in secret locations. Four hundred families had joined these troops, and they were demining land at the border and settling on it. The land had been allocated by an official in Phnom Penh, however there was potential for conflict with local authorities. The Commander estimated over two thirds of his soldiers didn't know how HIV spread and didn't use condoms. All STI drugs and condoms had stopped eight months ago after it was found they were selling them. There was a week's training two years ago for 20 men, presumably peer educators.

When I went back to see the Commander on the 20th May with the Director of the AIDS Program and the MSF educator, he was more forthcoming. Fifty men had died of AIDS last year. There were also another 6000 border troops, and they didn't have any current HIV/AIDS prevention and care programs. The men were continuing to die with four or five dead already this year and another four to five sick.

I spoke with Eap and the Provincial Director of Health, and they contacted NCHADS and the military in Phnom Penh. In late May I toured again with an Army Health Educator. By the time

I left FHI/Impact planned peer educator and condom programs. By 2002 70% of the military in Cambodia had peer educator programs and condoms, together with 25% of the police.

It was not only the military and border areas which were at risk, but areas where families were forced to migrate to Thailand or border areas. Arlys said her home care program Dhammayietra in Mongol Borei had 17 patients with AIDS who had been admitted in the previous four months. All of them had histories of migration. Village leaders estimated from thirty to seventy percent of the villagers migrated. There were many poor and landless people in that area, as the military had grabbed much of their land when the hostilities with the Khmer Rouge stopped two to three years earlier.

In 2019 the Cambodian Government, through the World Bank, began addressing the problem of landlessness. Over 5000 landless and land poor families were allocated 17,000 hectares of residential and farmland. Land titles were distributed to almost half of them. The project provided roads, tracks to rural plots, infrastructure for water supply, and accessible schools and health clinics.

After meeting the Commander on the 20th May the MSF educator, Director of the AIDS Program and I went to Boeung Trakoun. We met the Police Chief, the Village Chief, and the Health Chief. There were 1000 families in Boeung Trakoun, and the town had 15 brothel-based sex workers and 50 entertainment workers who sold sex from 10 karaoke bars. There were many patrons including the 30 to 300 Khmer daily labourers who worked in Thailand, 150 demobilised soldiers and the military from Thma Puok.

A few of the housewives also sold sex in Thailand while 80% of the adolescents were addicted to yama. There was also sexual trafficking. Small children wandered around sniffing glue, and there was gambling everywhere. There was a lot of work to do but the MSF Educator felt the situation was slowly improving.

That night we slept there in the NPA (Norwegian People's Aid) compound in Boeung Trakoun. People talked late into the night and then the alarm awoke us at 5am with a Khmer voice reading the news. I heard people washing and cars pulling out.

The MSF educator and I then left for a meeting with the Thais in Aran. We met Eap and he told us one of the NCHADS doctors said Cambodia was one of the three countries worldwide slowly turning the epidemic around. The others were Thailand and Uganda. I was surprised and moved, that despite all the problems, the nation was succeeding.

There were 20 Cambodians and 12 Thais in a flash hotel. The Thais wanted to support Cambodia to set up an organisation for People Living with AIDS. As we pointed out it was People dying with AIDS rather than living with it. There were few reliable HIV testing clinics and very few antiretrovirals, but we agreed.

The breakthrough came in 2003 when Cambodia received funding from the Global Fund for free antiretrovirals through its public health system. In 2004 and 2005 the number of patients receiving antiretrovirals increased from 2311 to 10,537 or 38% of those eligible for antiretrovirals so there were People living with AIDS. Almost forty percent of the patients who needed medication were receiving it. The continuum of care program was introduced and included voluntary testing and counselling, ART, TB care, HIV care, the prevention of mother to child transmission, and support groups for people living with AIDS.

———

Marie Charles, the author of an article, *HIV epidemic in Cambodia, one of the poorest countries in Southeast Asia, a success story* said the Director of NCHADS Dr Mean Chi Vun, was responsible for the turnaround of HIV/AIDS in Cambodia, with his vision for sustainable long-term delivery, and a national strategy.

She described curbing an HIV epidemic as solving a large puzzle. But all the pieces needed to be put together at the same time. Otherwise, the groups that were still at risk could reinfect the others. That's why it was necessary to address the gap in services to the military and the border areas. NCHADS did that promptly when alerted, but we needed to be on the ground to identify it.

From thinking about the problem on a macro scale I returned to the micro. In Aran after the meeting, I saw a small boy standing by the money changer. They told him to go. He looked so thin and sad, I bought him milk, fish and peanuts.

———

On Wednesday the 9th of May before going to work, sitting on my veranda I listened to the clop of a horse drawn cart and the chuckle of a lizard. Yesterday I'd looked at a lizard in the garden, and realised that magnified a million times, it would look like a dinosaur. It was these moments of awareness and relaxation that enabled me to keep going.

I had meetings all day including with Tess from FHI. We felt more confident about Poipet because the USAID money had come through. But it was still unsafe up there. She told me four people were killed in a daytime robbery.

I asked my language tutor about a Khmer man with two-inch-long fingernails. He grew them to show he didn't work in the fields. We discussed the conditions for those landless people who did. The owner supplied fertiliser and tools, and the farmer got one third of the profit.

On Thursday we continued with the situation analysis and discussed abortions. As the driver on my way to Pailin, had pointed out, the lack of contraception and the consequent abortions were a problem. It was the lack of the availability of contraception that contributed to the number of unwanted children. I had been to the Marie Stopes clinic in Battambang and was impressed by the efficiency and cleanliness of the clinic, but it was a world away from Poipet, Pailin, Malai and the border villages.

There are now more services for the rural areas. Marie Stopes in their Cambodian website in 2023 advertised Marie Stopes ladies, midwives and doctors were able to provide services in rural areas. Another pro-choice organisation, MSI, mentions self-managed abortion for pregnancies up to three months on their website. In our situation analysis we acknowledged the problem and suggested a women's clinic be provided.

We then discussed homosexuality. I struggled to explain this to some of my Khmer counterparts. STI clinic and NGO staff received anecdotal information that groups of men from Sisophon hired high school boys to have sex with them at parties in Poipet. It may have occurred in prisons and wats . The MSF Director had visited prisons and had provided condoms to those who had STI symptoms. She said she just provided a few as some prisoners had tried to choke themselves to death on them. Homosexuality was not widely discussed in Cambodia at that time and young men were often unaware of it. It was a vulnerable group. An FHI report from 2000 in Phnom Penh identified that of the men who had sex with men surveyed, 26% had an STI and 14% were HIV positive.

By Saturday 12th May I was exhausted and instead of doing the housework reflected on the people I worked with. One of the NGO workers had lost all his family, as had his wife, during Pol Pot's time.

These people are amazing. They have lost so much and understand they need to live well. They are authentic and need and give affection. If they like you, they tell you. Life is too short and too precious to lie or pretend.

In the photos taken I look tough and brown, and slightly wizened. The Angkor Wat photos were different. I was on holiday then and looking after myself mentally and physically. I still had to learn not to drive myself too hard.

The 8000 underserviced soldiers at the border had been reported to the Director of Health and NCHADS, but now I had to get back to Thma Puok, We needed to keep working. As well as reporting risks, we had to slow them.

Chapter Sixteen

MARGINALISED WOMEN AND CHILDREN – JUNE 2001

I now had a leave date, 23rd July, three months away, but there was still a lot of work to do. Vulnerable populations and places, including the military and Poipet, were still not getting the assistance they needed. I also needed to continue working on the Thma Puok project and complete a situation analysis with the technical working group.

I left early on Monday May 14th for Thma Puok. The day before it had rained heavily and the lowlands near Sisophon were flooded. As we turned off to the uplands a sower was scattering seed and people were ploughing, the plough between two yoked oxen, the furrow slicing the earth. Motorbikes with trailers were towing trailers with four large water jars. Five was too many. The driver had seen a trailer with five overturn. They traded the water for rice.

We had a District AIDS meeting with police, military, teachers, KBA (The Khmer Buddhist Association), and NPA (Norwegian People's Aid). Besides preventative programs we discussed providing support and training to the staff in the six private pharmacies, particularly that owned by the nurse. Another problem discussed was the lack of care from the health clinic. They did not provide symptomatic or Level A care for mobile patients including Bactrim to prevent pneumonia. The staff were untrained and there were no guidelines.

As the situation analysis pointed out, there were no national guidelines for providing symptomatic level A treatment to mobile patients, including those with diarrhoea, skin problems and pain. Some NGOs, such as MSF developed their own protocols. Arlys developed guidelines for her home care program, including district hospital referral for all patients with oesophageal thrush. Towards the end of June there was a five-day provincial workshop for care of AIDS patients which I participated in. However, the drugs were not scheduled to arrive until the end of the year.

When I returned to Sisophon I said goodbye to Edith at a farewell lunch. She was a good friend and I missed her during the last couple of months.

Before work on Wednesday, I picked my way through the mud to my road. The little orchard was green, and the mountain behind it partly covered in mist. I ran towards it pretending it was Mt Barney near Brisbane. I slept with a rock from Barney under my pillow. At the market I bought an extra blanket for Bo and watched small boys in white shirts and blue shorts from the Chinese school trying to push their school bus out of the mud.

We continued with the situation analysis in relation to gender issues. The national survey of 15,000 women in 2000 showed the depth of the gender gap in Banteay Meanchey, one of the least developed provinces. This was not only in relation to men, but women from other provinces.

While half of the women in Banteay Meanchey couldn't read, over 90 percent of women in Phnom Penh could. More than a third of women in Banteay Meanchey hadn't been to school and half believed it was more important to educate boys than girls. More than half of the women in Banteay Meanchey believed a woman shouldn't work outside the home and the family rice-fields. Almost 90 percent of the Banteay Meanchey women had no knowledge of their legal rights in relation to in relation to marriage, violence and labour, yet 1 in 6 women throughout Cambodia experienced sexual violence.

In the situation analysis we included women's lack of protection by law and law enforcement groups, their inability to negotiate condom use and choices about sex, and the high rate of domestic violence. We suggested police, women's affairs, and women's NGOS collaborate on cases of rape and domestic violence, and that legal advice be provided. Female police could assist with domestic violence cases, and health staff be trained to deal effectively and confidentially with such cases.

We also advocated men's addictions, including gambling, drunkenness, drug use and use of sex workers, be addressed using male focus groups and elders. Youth with addictions, could also consider this model. It was suggested gender issues be included in the school curriculum.

Research about domestic violence was carried out in 2015 in rural communities around Siem Reap. Rice wine was cheap and widely available. There was alcohol related violence during festivals and community events, both in public places and family settings. There were also more motorcycle crashes, and pedestrians on poorly lit village roads were more vulnerable.

Children were encouraged to drink alcohol early, and there were no age restrictions. Some people spent their income on alcohol rather than food and education. Drunkenness encouraged high risk sexual behaviour particularly in karaoke bars. Law enforcement was weak and there were no support services to help people address the problem. It was suggested community-based leaders and networks organise community events and training. Nationally, other considerations included limiting youth access to alcohol, strengthened law enforcement and responsible service delivery.

Two days later, on Friday 18th May I was at the Poipet market when a woman came up with a cage. I was horrified when she whipped the cloth away revealing a beautiful green parrot. I then met Tess from FHI. She now had access to all six casinos, and we started our round including their massage parlours and karaoke rooms. One massage parlour was like a brightly lit fishbowl, with lounging, bored girls and one way glass. There was a tall, buxom, slightly grey-haired madam in tight trousers. She looked a little embarrassed but was polite and deferential. The casinos provided free food to entice clients to keep gambling. Tess was impressive and the staff accepted her.

Out in the muddy streets was a man in a cart. Both his legs had been blown off. We toured the shacks and brothels. Many businesses had guards, and there was a bed in the guardroom often used for sex. Late at night we were back at the hotel. It had a very noisy air conditioner, a door which wouldn't shut, no water, no toilet paper and yet it was full.

It was a relief to have a break in Aran on Saturday with Arlys, and then on Sunday the 20th I rushed back to Sisophon. We held a candlelight memorial with monks and candles for those who had died of AIDS. It was a worldwide event, and a service was held in Phnom Penh.

That day I also met an American nurse, who worked in the Safety and Surveillance Working Group funded by GAVI, to improve the quality and quantity of drugs available in developing countries. There was $US35 million available for two of the seven countries investigated. She said it was unlikely Cambodia would be chosen because their research with tracer drugs showed there were many fake drugs.

On Monday the MSF educator and I went back to Thma Puok in the MSF cruiser. The rice fields were a luminous green, and there were puffy white clouds in a very blue sky. People with a yoke across their shoulders and a pair of buckets, carried water between the fields, while a few were still ploughing. Oxen grazed on the vast plane. At times the cruiser ploughed through water, up to the bonnet, and we rescued a blue truck that was stuck.

We called in at Thma Puok to see the District Governor. He looked tired. We discussed the training of 42 village chiefs. The District AIDS Office (DAO) staff had designed a two-day and a half day program for them, including a morning on STIs. He wanted me to take it. We picked up the DAO staff and drove to Boeung Trakoun. When we arrived, it was tense. A high-ranking soldier had sold cows worth over $A 60,000 to a Thai middleman who hadn't paid. The Cambodians raided his house, kidnapped his wife, and hid her in the forest. There was concern fighting would break out, but both sides were negotiating.

Later I spoke with the AusAID Agricultural Advisor. He said there were rules for selling cows including obtaining vaccinations and the Thais were aware of them. There was also a dengue outbreak which occurred annually after the rains. The villagers were given an insecticide, Abate, to prevent mosquito breeding in the water jars and advised to get rid of possible breeding sites. Two or three children were sick in most communities.

At a brothel a drunken sex worker told us she'd tested HIV positive from a private laboratory and neither of her two boyfriends wore condoms. It was difficult to have a coherent conversation with her, but we spoke with the brothel owner. Then we toured the pharmacies. There was one run by a solider , very well stocked and we suspected the supplies had been stolen. We watched the bored workers in another sorting out pills for sciatica, a common complaint, after the constant stooping in the rice-fields and the damp of the wet. We ate protected animal for lunch, probably crocodile, then spoke with some chiefs about the training. They said they were busy planting rice but would attend when they'd finished.

On the second day the Director of the District AIDS Office and I went to see the Commander, then had a meeting with KBA. They planned to carry out a home care program in Thma Puok. I was concerned about support from the clinic, however they established a program and by 2003 provided support for 35 people living with HIV/AIDS and 133 children affected by AIDS.

They also helped patients access medical care, as was clear by their support of a widow with 4 children aged from 4 to 14. Her husband had died of AIDS four years earlier and she was sick. While she and her 14-year-old son grew vegetables, her 9-year-old son looked after the two smallest children. When they ran out of money they slept in the forest. She and the two eldest children worked illegally in Thailand and sometimes they were caught. The daily income they made (max $1.5) was never enough to feed them and buy medicine.

KBA began working with the family in 2002. They gave her US$7, and she paid US$10 for a small plot of land with a house. The two eldest children were supported to attend school, and she and her youngest child (also HIV positive) received treatment for their opportunistic infections. Her 18-year-old daughter then returned to live with them.

On Friday I had difficulty getting the protocol right to contact the military hierarchy. I drafted a letter, which the Director of Health checked. He redrafted it. Then I followed up to check we had the wording right and had sent it to the right person. By the end of the day, we knew a representative from the military would arrive in the next few days.

———·———

Saturday 26th May was busy, but in a different way. First, I met the UNICEF consultant's friend, also a consultant, a coloured woman , clever, capable, and confident but very lonely. There was a lot of prejudice in Cambodia then against coloured people . The Khmers, particularly the women, used whitening powder and tried to keep out of the sun. At least with myself and the consultant who had rented my top floor, she could feel at home. Then Eap arrived to advise me that NCHADS wanted four to five more District AIDS Committees formed as money was available from the Asian Development Bank. In the evening Bo told me about the three hectares of land his mother-law had gifted them. At last, the family could live off their own rice. He had hired a tractor and ploughed the land and now was ready to plant.

———·———

By Wednesday the military health educator had arrived, and with a colleague from the Health Department, we went to meet a General and his health team in Malai. The health educator talked incessantly, explained things clearly, and was funny and interesting. As we travelled, we discussed monkeys, cows and then horses. He told me a very senior military advisor would tour in June and I was grateful.

As we travelled on the road to Poipet I watched the road building. Teams of women with blankets, their faces covered by kramas or checked cotton scarves, laid heavy rocks on the road, and covered them with blankets. A roller rolled over the blankets, and the process was repeated with gravel. A tar machine covered with black pitch, belched black smoke while a man tinkered with it. It wasn't a permanent fix and after every wet season it had to be redone.

On the road to Malai we agreed focus group discussions were a good strategy. Many soldiers were aware of how HIV spread and had friends who had died, but behaviour change was still a problem. Alcohol consumption, peer pressure, availability of condoms and STI treatment were factors.

We met the General's medical assistant and toured with him. Out of 2000 soldiers 50 died last year, while in one battalion of 370 soldiers five men had died. We were taken to see a dying 24-year-old. Four friends surrounded him, boiling a large pot of roots. How different it was from the General I saw dying in Sisophon with his wife in attendance. His friends accepted his death, and knew they were not at risk from him. They did not expect a miracle. I hoped they would protect themselves.

We then went for lunch with the General in his expensive car. He believed in discipline and the leader setting an example. He said yama was a problem but didn't believe AIDS was. I was grateful we had met his medical assistant beforehand. I was worried about the lunch because I often paid and my funds were low, but he paid. The food was great, and the four soldiers drank a bottle of brandy between them. I managed to persuade our driver not to drink too much.

On the 2nd of June, my birthday, I had a party on a roof in Battambang. It was the liveliest in my life. We had a band who did seven numbers including the Battambang Blues. There were many people including a deminer talking about Kosovo, one of my Khmer colleagues talking about a business collapse, a consultant from IOM and the AusAID Agricultural Advisor. He had worked in PNG in the seventies. There were resources but they were poorly managed. He said Cambodia was difficult because of the different culture, loneliness, the lack of recreation, services, roads, rubbish, and poor health services.

There were candles, fairy lights and African music. I enjoyed dancing to the strong proud, passionate, yet sad voices of African women. They were singing for all women; the women of Cambodia, the women in Poipet, the sex workers, the women facing AIDS, singing for the whole sadness of the place. I got home at 1am.

By Sunday I was in Phnom Penh. Despite my fears it was a good trip. I paid 650 baht for the whole front seat and got there comfortably at 2pm. It was noisy at the backpackers, so I shifted closer to the Mekong River.

On Monday, the 4th June I met Graham Fordham, the female AusAID consultant's replacement. He was a social anthropologist with ten years of HIV experience in Thailand. He described Thai society as complex. They had studied the west for the past three to four hundred years and decided what to adopt. They were consummate politicians and had a sense of superiority.

Graham confirmed there was a lack of services for young people between 14 and 19 years in Cambodia. No behaviour surveillance has been carried out and yet some were sexually active. They represented 17% of those who had abortions. He also felt girls needed to stay in school until they were 14, so they had the skills to look after themselves and the children they would bear.

In the provincial situation analysis, the technical working group had declared 'The problems of youth are not being addressed.' It was noted no behavioural surveillance or surveillance had been carried out, there were no youth friendly reproductive health services, no safe recreational activities, and no peer educator programs. We advocated that a youth advisor be employed to work with working groups, the department of Education, increase skills in service providers and carry out research.

Graham published Adolescent and Youth Reproductive Health in Cambodia, in January 2003. He advocated a policy be designed, research be carried out, NGOs participate in interagency working groups, suitable visual media be developed and the capacity of public servants in ministries be developed.

———

On Tuesday the 5th I woke up at 6am. It was already light. Down at the Mekong the great river was brilliant in the sun, with sampans, a tiny cabin in front, a solitary upright figure at the back paddling with a single oar. There were youths sleeping on the embankment and although the Chinese tai chi class had finished there were a few pairs of women languidly batting a shuttlecock. An old Chinese man, stripped to the waist was practising his Bruce Lee moves while others were walking briskly up and down the esplanade. There were cages of sparrows waiting to be freed, a few people selling fish, a few police with batons giving orders and a pile of dirt being shifted by labourers.

Before I arrived, while I was holidaying in NZ, I had listened to talkback radio. A recently returned volunteer from Africa mourned the lack of cows in downtown Wellington. I'm going to be just the same about this place, I thought.

Later speaking with the head of the Cambodian Red Cross I found the Deputy Director of Health had become their Vice President. She was delighted.

One of the nicest complements I got while I was in Cambodia was from the WHO Country Director who said Banteay Meanchey had become a different place. Everyone was proud of themselves, and everyone was working.

I had fun discussing youth services in Boeung Trakoun with the UNICEF consultant. He proposed summer camp. I advised that these adolescent males sniffed glue, took yama, smuggled goods and frequented brothels. We compromised with the boxing club which the local policeman was asking for. NGOs were exploring the integration of credit schemes for those families living with AIDS. USAID money was going to KHANA, to CARE and FHI and the military were beginning to secure support.

My last discussion was about Koh Kong, a border province with Vietnam and the increase in injecting drug users. It was estimated in a survey carried out in Phnom Penh that injection of drugs had increased from 0.6% of all drug use in 2000 to 10% in 2004. In 2004 HIV prevalence in people who injected drugs was estimated to be between 14 to 31 %, compared with 3% to 18% amongst noninjecting drug users. There were an estimated 1,750 injecting drug users. Risks included 40 % of the injecting drug users having multiple sex partners and rarely using condoms, while 47% sold blood and shared needles.

By 2008 there were 14 state run drug treatment and rehabilitation centres catering for from 100 to 200 clients In Banteay Meanchey there were two, one run by the Military Police and another by the Ministry of Social Affairs, Veterans, and Youth Rehabilitation.

Banteay Meanchey also took a community approach. In 2010 the province held its first community-based drug dependence and treatment workshop. It was a five-day training session for health workers in primary care centres, referral hospitals; and NGO workers who worked with injecting drug users. Over 200 people attended the workshop sponsored by UNODC (United Nations Office on Drugs and Crime). It was conducted by the International Network of Treatment and Rehabilitation Centres (Treatnet). Follow up workshops were held. It was a community-based solution in the way home based care programs had been.

That was the last time I went to Phnom Penh. I said goodbye in the same way I had said hello. By watching the sunrise over the Mekong. Four young men on a sampan were silhouetted against the sunrise as they slowly pulled up their nets. The sun light glittered on the water. Thirty or forty young men jogged past me and the Tai Chi group with their deliberate graceful gestures. Nearby a dishevelled young man prayed to Buddha and burnt incense. A trim long-haired blonde ran past. Coming back, I passed the coffin shop, a woman squatting sorting out root vegetables, the hotel with the sign the Royal Hiness, and the shop called Nick Neek.

I thought of my hunger to belong and share the burden. I had become part of the life here in a way I had never imagined. I was going to miss this country, these people. I'd given it everything and now I was burnt out. Others had taken over and I needed to rediscover myself in my own family, my own culture.

Chapter Seventeen

BOEING TRAKOUN TRANSFORMED
& DEPARTURE – JULY 2001

On Monday 11th June I took the boat to Siem Reap where I'd been invited to a conference with the Thais. The cabin was very crowded, but I was happy to sit on the roof. Although I got sunburnt, visions of overloaded boats sinking in the developing world kept me there, together with the view.

We passed huts on the land, and huts on stilts in the water with people fishing. From the bank children waved, women did their washing and then we passed a school. The children rushed down the bank waved to us and then climbed back. A herd of cows came down to drink. I saw one man fishing and near him a puff of smoke. He was dynamiting.

Then I dozed. The bell rang a few times and when I looked up all I could see was the vast expanse of the Tonle Sap, the inland sea and sky merging and above low clouds.

There was no wharf, so the anchor was dropped, and we were ferried in. I enjoyed the ride through a floating village, past floating hulks, a floating school, perhaps the school the UNICEF consultant and I had worked on, and a floating clinic. Pigs floated by on an old barge with a few trees on it. People were cooking and I was near enough to see their faces. Many of them looked miserable. Then we followed a canal, the banks eroded by the constant wash of canoes, and finally waded ashore where the waiting touts tried to kidnap us for various guest houses.

I woke up on Tuesday with a mouse nibbling me, so I put a sock in its hole. Early morning, and there were four street boys sleeping in a heap on the pavement and a couple who looked very thin. The tourist income obviously wasn't trickling down to them. Meeting again today.

Wednesday 13th June and I was back in Sisophon after a painful trip. I paid an extra $US10 to get the truck going when it broke down and then we were held up at a bridge for two hours. The villagers had removed the boards and when the waiting drivers lost patience, invited them to pay to proceed. I finally arrived at 4pm and discovered a huge electricity bill, US$70 for the month, and I wasn't there.

The next day I found out why the bill was so large. The neighbour had reconnected to my line and recommenced building renovations. The news from the office was more cheerful.

The European Union was going to support an STI clinic and men who have sex with men. MSF was leaving Banteay Meanchey, but CARE would employ their local staff and the Director would hand the library over to them. The Reproductive Health Association (RHAC) would support clinics, high risk groups and indirect sex workers, or those who didn't work out of brothels. The Cambodian Family Development Service (CFDS) would continue to support programs for people and families living with HIV/

AIDS. Family Health International would continue to organise the monthly strategic meeting in Poipet. The Cambodian Red Cross (CRC) would work with Police and finally the Social Environment Agricultural Development Organisation (SEADO) and CRC would do more work with schools.

On Saturday I went to see Sarin. Her husband wanted to begin a tourist business in Siem Reap with a partner. To support the family, she needed to work again. She was thinking of working in Poipet with Corinne for ZOA but would need accommodation.

On Monday 18th, the landlord said he would provide me with a new electricity connection. Before the neighbour connected to my line, my monthly bill was $US30 to $US40 and I could afford to run the fridge and even make yoghurt.

——·——

On Thursday 21st of June I went up to Boeung Trakoun with the WHO Doctor. We couldn't stay overnight as we couldn't get a security pass from the UN. With us were the Director of the Thma Puok District AIDS program and his deputy. On the way up there were two spots where the villagers had partly dismantled the bridges and asked for bribes before allowing traffic through. At one spot the road went through the river. The driver drove down and out into the flooded rice fields and got stuck. The WHO Doctor took over. They dug out the wheels, put rocks under them and he got the land cruiser out.

At the clinic there was confusion about a possible cholera outbreak. The doctor asked them to report it to NPA headquarters, the provincial health authorities and WHO. There was a discussion about dengue. NPA said they had referred thirty dengue cases to the Health Centre who reported receiving just one. Some people had difficulty accessing the clinic which was some distance from the town. Some of the districts reported they had not received Abate sent to eradicate the mosquito larva in water containers. Two children had died of dengue on their way to Thai hospitals. The hospital at Thma Puok had treated children with dengue and saved one child's life with a blood transfusion.

We visited the brothels. The sex workers were seen by the District AIDS Officers every month and were now using condoms and attending STI clinics. The health centre also included partner tracing in its follow-up. More condoms were being sold, and the barber said he used a new blade for each client. The village chief enjoyed the AIDS training he attended, and we said we would send him AIDS awareness videos for the karaoke bars and boxing club. The boxing club was thriving. We had learnt from this pilot project and hoped similar projects could be run in other districts.

———

By Friday I was very tired, hardly slept at all and had a slightly itchy throat. Bo was upset too. His one-year-old son has been vomiting and had diarrhoea for three days. He took him to a doctor who prescribed medication, which cost him $US60, a good chunk of his monthly salary. We found out three days later he had dengue but thankfully he didn't get too sick. It was different with one of the two expatriates who got it. He had to be evacuated to Singapore.

I saw Arlys on Saturday 23rd June, and she told me about a woman in Svay Chek who bled during delivery and presented to the referral hospital. A doctor went to the market, bought some packed cells for 1000 baht, admitted her, and saved her life.

Haemorrhage during and after childbirth was one of the three major reasons why the maternal mortality rate in Cambodia was so high, 437 maternal deaths per 100,000 live births. The other two causes were eclampsia and deaths following abortions.

Arlys also told me about a miliary man in his thirties who was HIV positive. He was married for the third time and still healthy. He decided he would die, gathered his brothers and sisters together, told them, and was dead within a month. We agreed our role was to support people living with HIV/AIDS, with whatever they wanted.

I thought about the peace of Arlys house. It was on a quiet street next to a lagoon, and she looked over trees. She was leaving soon for a break and said she would be sorry to come back in August and find me gone.

My house mate on the top floor was packing and because she had no time during the day she packed at night, finally stopping at midnight.

I spoke at an AIDS care workshop on Monday 25th June. It ran for five days and provided practical training. It would be six months before the drugs came through. Finally, the health staff were being trained, protocols provided and in six months would have the drugs they needed.

I walked to work the next day as the motorbike wouldn't start. A siren sounded, not for an ambulance but a pickup, the tray packed with back-to-back gendarmes, the barrels of their rifles against their chests. This was the Governor's Army. As I'd seen them on my first working day in Sisophon, so I saw them on one of my last.

The house was quiet. My housemate had left.

I went to a big party, my last in the country. The former CARERE Director, the man who took me in and supported me, was there. We said goodbye. He was a good man and understood how I felt about going home. There were strange things to eat, tongue, intestines, and large chunks of steak and chicken. I preferred the pancakes.

At work Eap told me there was $650 million from donors for HIV/AIDS this year, or $72 million more than last year. USAID has given money at a government-to-government level directly for AIDS. It was $US9 million and for just a few provinces.

I heard Sarin had a job with ZOA working in the Poipet Health Centre with government staff. It would be very demanding, but I knew if anyone could do it, she could. She was looking for a house in Poipet.

———

On Thursday 28th June I was asked to accompany a young Japanese

IOM (International Organisation for Migration) consultant, on an overnight visit to Poipet. IOM was developing a proposal for the Burmese border which included support for the primary health care system. The Thais had requested IOM consider a similar project at Poipet.

We talked non-stop for two days. The consultant was a good interviewer, very perceptive and asked searching questions. She confirmed there were now more boys trafficked than girls in Poipet. They suspected the number of paedophile rings in Thailand had grown, fuelled by the internet.

I was picked up by a black taxi and we drove towards the black sky over Poipet. Arriving we alighted into a sea of mud outside the SEADO office (Social Environment Agricultural Development Organisation). We met Tess from FHI and toured the casinos. The consultant was shocked Cambodians were not allowed to gamble.

We stayed at the best hotel, the Poipet Pass. It was a square concrete block, set back from the road and surrounded by karaoke rooms full of heavily made-up girls. In the lobby a smart self-assured young man told us we were late, and he had let out one of the rooms. We were shown a room with a very large double bed. We both felt that was taking intimacy too far and I asked for a camp bed. They found one, together with a cubicle under the stairs.

We went out to eat, talked a long time and came back to the room which now had mosquitoes. I had a long hot shower before going down to my bunker. I went to sleep despite the karaoke. The all-night barking dogs of Sisophon had toughened me up. I woke at six thirty, and by seven we were at the border. The consultant watched streams of people crossing illegally into Thailand in view of the police and the customs officers. Some children carried black bundles of clothes for the Thai markets. By 8am the stream was lighter, and people made way for the cargo haulers.

After breakfast we went to SEADO. A peer educator was working with volunteers using the HIV/AIDS manual designed by FHI. Tess said it was critical to find out first what people knew and believed, and work from there. We then stopped at the MSF sexual health clinic. There were around thirty sex workers learning Thai. Some looked about thirteen. They came each day because they said it gave them hope. They had a respectful male teacher.

The consultant then told me about the garment factories. There were over hundred in Cambodia and CARE worked in five. The workers were often country girls, and naïve. CARE supported workers by arranging events, including karaoke and dancing and held condom awareness and distribution sessions.

After lunch we were driven to the resettlement areas, with small houses and gardens, and saw the other vast tracts of land owned by the military. Corinne told us how difficult life was for people here, those who had been relocated after being evicted, and those in the small houses we had seen. The consultant then went to the IOM transit centre, where there were 15 boys and some Vietnamese. She said it was difficult to speak with them about HIV/AIDS prevention when they didn't know where they would eat or sleep that night. There was a big meeting with the Thais, and we got back to Battambang on Saturday.

Before I left, I wondered whether we had made an impact in Poipet. There was an improvement in services, and political engagement including the formation of a Poipet District AIDS

Committee with the Third Deputy Governor, but it wasn't until December 2005 they got what they needed. It was then the US Ambassador opened an HIV/AIDS testing and treatment clinic. In 16 months, they provided treatment to 666 HIV infected patients including 310 who received antiretroviral treatment Besides an HIV in-patient unit, health staff were trained, laboratory equipment and reagents provided, an isolation unit built for AIDS patients with TB, an X Ray machine provided, meals provided to patients, and the maternity wing upgraded.

Indeed, USAID transformed the services in Banteay Meanchey Province as I had hoped. They spent US $ 1. 5 million in Banteay Meanchey Province from 2002 to 2007. This included a budget for three HIV clinics. The first opened in Sisophon in December 2004, the second in Mongol Borei in June 2005, and the last in Poipet in December 2005. These clinics provided ART and dropped the mortality rates by half. In 2004 before the introduction of ART, 37 % of HIV infected TB patients died during TB treatment compared to 5% of patients with TB only. In 2005 after the introduction of ART, 18% of HIV infected TB patients died.

I stayed in Battambang as I had meetings with the Provincial AIDS Program staff, the military, and women's affairs for final reports. When I attended the meetings on Monday, I was surprised to learn from the Provincial AIDS staff that up to half of the soldiers were not wearing condoms in brothels. Instead, they showed the sex workers a certificate which stated they were HIV negative. I wondered aloud how members of the 100% condom monitoring group would respond to that and raised it with the Director of Health.

The Women's Affairs PAS representative had held workshops for 160 women in 4 villages. I told her I was about to travel to Kampong Chhnang to hand over Women's Affairs to another Australian volunteer working there.

On Wednesday 4th July I arrived in Kampong Chhnang on the Tonle Sap, just 90 km from Phnom Penh. I had a rugged journey down in a pickup, jammed in the front seat with a woman and her small child. It was my fault as I had only paid US$5 for a single place, instead of US$10 for the full seat.

The volunteer worked part-time with the Ministry of Women's Affairs with HIV/AIDS. She had previously worked in Cambodia for seven years as a midwifery trainer. Another volunteer also worked for the Ministry of Women's Affairs but hadn't found it very interesting. That changed after the big floods last year, the worst in 40 years. They affected 56. 000 hectares of rice fields, and 17,000 families were short of rice. Over 100 people died, and houses, roads and wells were destroyed.

The volunteer went round the villages and asked what they wanted. She applied to AusAID for a project to provide rice and vegetable seeds and training to 30 to 40 villages, including climate preparedness, and the construction of 30 to 40 wells and toilets. The $US200,000 proposal was successful, and she bought 127 tons of rice seed and vegetables, distributed it, and provided funds for 50 toilets and wells. The toilets were not built in villages next to the river. These were prone to flooding ten months of the year, and the wells were built above the flood level. She was also going to include HIV/AIDS awareness programs. Both women said Kampong Chunnang was vulnerable as it was on the main truck route to Vietnam. There was no 100% condom program, but FHI provided support to sex workers.

———·———

Back in Sisophon I went to an NGO meeting on Wednesday morning 11th July chaired by the Chairman of the local NGO network and head of SEADO (Social Environmental Agricultural Development Organisation). He had attended a ten-day workshop run by KHANA which supported local NGOs to carry out HIV prevention and care projects.. He had carried out a needs analysis and had $US 14,000 for working in six villages. A KHANA representative would visit Banteay Meanchey and introduce them to Arlys. The results of the USAID support for KHANA would soon improve education and support in the villages.

———·———

In the evening my language teacher arrived. He had just returned from a four-day workshop in Battambang about child centred learning. He told me books sent to schools sometimes ended up in private bookshops. I wrote my name in my diary and above it he wrote my name in Khmer.

I slept better than usual on Thursday, and on Friday morning walking up the hill, I watched a woman chipping rocks from a large pile beside her. Her children were beside her, then disappeared into their shack. Others were heaving boulders down the hill, and at the bottom small boys loaded the smashed rocks into a cart drawn by a tractor.

I went to a barbecue with the Swedish deminer who leased Edith's house. He trained dogs to sniff them out mines. He served big hunks of barbecued beef, and I came home and ate porridge.

On Sunday I had lunch with Sarin and her family in the restaurant on the way to Battambang. We ate on platforms in the lagoon and watched the fish gulping, from lack of oxygen. We threw fish feed in, but they didn't rise. Sarin told me about her job at Poipet Health Centre. On Friday she and the health centre chief ran out to a pregnant woman who had fainted outside with heavy vaginal bleeding. They inserted four IVs, and Sarin bought some packed red cells and paid for blood to be cross matched at the Mongol Borei Hospital. On Saturday she went to the hospital and found the woman had not arrived. She had died in the ambulance. Sarin was very upset. She planned to carry out outreach activities with her team and said she would give the job three months and reassess.

———

I was back in Boeung Trakoun on Monday 16th July with the Director of the Thma Puok District AIDS program and his deputy. We were at the brothels and one of the sex workers, a tall angular girl, was wearing a dark blue tee shirt with the words 'Just do me now.' Another girl was very delicately picking out the fish from a soup. There was a spat, and then it was the tall girl in the tee shirt who had the fish soup. The madam with the round face and slightly glazed eyes told me the girls made lots of money and went on to get married and have children. I protested as I knew many of these girls were in permanent debt to the brothel owner. The Director said some of the girls were from the country and could return to their villages. I hoped so.

In Aran on the 18th July, Wednesday it was so quiet I couldn't sleep. There were no barking dogs, no noisy funerals, no traffic starting at 4.30am. I met Arlys who said her team had become more confident in the few weeks she was away, and she felt her absence was productive. They were learning. I agreed an interrupted presence was preferable as it gave people autonomy. Arlys was pleased we had applied for a six-week scholarship for Eap in Japan. We said goodbye as she was going on leave.

21st July Saturday and my last weekend in Sisophon. It was raining and very muddy. In the afternoon the rain cleared, and I went to see the WHO doctor. We discussed the health centre volunteers. It was important they knew how HIV/AIDS was spread and how to provide simple care. It helped prevent patients and families spending vast amounts on traditional healers, or fake or inappropriate drugs.

On Saturday night there were so many dogs barking over-night it was like an orchestra. Surprisingly I enjoyed it. On Sunday I worked all day.

The next week on Monday I went up to Thma Puok with a government official We tried to take a taxi up to Thma Puok as there was no room in the MSF vehicle. However, they had video game equipment in the back and couldn't leave because they wouldn't pay a police bribe. Finally, a friend of my companion took us both on his motorbike. Luckily my companion was just 47kg and me 65.

I slewed around on the back a fair bit and the drive through the mud seemed interminable. There were a couple of times I thought the driver had lost control, but I was wrong. Dawn, clear, limpid pale-yellow. Far away a tree was waving in the unseen wind. A flock of noisy parrots flew over. How magnificent this country must have been when it was forested. When we arrived, we had a cup of coffee to recover and then there were the meetings.

The wooden MSF house was full of memories, of people who had left including the doctor. I didn't go for a final walk, didn't go to the wat to gaze across the water and look at the spirit houses. I was tired. I spoke with the new MSF doctor who worked most of the time and had little personal life. It was as the AusAID Agricultural Advisor described, lonely. That was my last trip, and we consolidated the financial arrangements. The District Governor agreed the funds would go through their system and be withdrawn by voucher.

Arriving back on Tuesday 24th July, I had a meal with the AusAID Agricultural Advisor. He suggested I give Eap a reference and get a Khmer reference, and I did. The donors would watch the distribution of money, and if there were problems, control it from Phnom Penh.

I said goodbye to Geoff Manthey, the UNAIDS Director. He thanked me. He knew how rough it had been in Sisophon. He thought I'd saved hundreds, possibly thousands of lives.

I learned too the police charged each sex worker 1000 baht a month to continue operating. As the sex workers made around 50 baht a time it took them 20 sessions to pay off. At the last Provincial AIDS Committee meeting the Third Deputy Governor said they were to stop, and my counterpart Eap was determined they would.

My language teacher talked about his four daughters aged from 8 to 15 and in grades 3 to 8. At their school the parents paid 1 to 2 baht a day to supplement teachers' salaries. It was an honest system and they got homework. Both examples showed that despite the corruption, good people around me knew how to work with the system and achieve good outcomes.

For my simple farewell at the house, we had Pringles and Coca Cola and I had a shandy. Neither Bo nor my language teacher drank. When I returned, I missed them as I missed Sarin and Eap and so many of the people I had lived and worked with.

The next day I left for Thailand and stopped over at Aran.

I slept through the night, the first time I'd done so for months.

I then had a holiday in Thailand and Laos for a month and arrived back in Australia on the 22nd of August 2001.

Postscript

It was much harder to return than it was to go. I had been worried about returning and I was right. It was a crash landing. Not only was I physically, mentally, and spiritually exhausted, but I was grieving for Cambodia and my Cambodian family and friends. Not only had I lost them, but I had lost meaning and purpose. After facing daily life and death decisions, my biggest concern was whether I needed to drive into the village to get more groceries.

I cheered up briefly when I flew to the Asian Pacific International AIDS Conference in Melbourne in October and with Eap, was one of the presenters. I was thanked by a Cambodian Princess. Later at Peter Dutton's office I was presented with a certificate from the Government of Australia that acknowledged the work I had done in Cambodia.

Unlike the Solomons I have little desire to return to Cambodia, although in 2023, 5.45 million other tourists visited Cambodia and perhaps that's why. Twenty years ago, in Siem Reap I struggled with the crowds of tourists. Now there would be more, and billions of dollars of Chinese aid/investment appear to have McDonaldized parts of the country.

However, the government did a remarkable job reducing

poverty. Whereas 40 % of the population was under the poverty line in 2009 this dropped by more than half to 18% in 2020. The World Bank said this was because of stability and good economic management, with Cambodian workers moving from agriculture to manufacturing and services, with urban areas growing. In 2022, GDP per capita for Cambodia was US 1760 dollars, up from 364 dollars in 2003.The average world GDP per capita was US$12,600 in 2022. Average life expectancy increased from 59 in 2000 to 71.5 in 2024.

The lack of safe water, sanitation and reliable electricity were major concerns in 2000 but that has changed. Cambodia has been one of the fastest countries to electrify in the world as it expanded energy access from 6.6 % of the population to 97.5 % by the end of 2021. There were just 350 villages without power in early 2022. Clean water and sanitation coverage now reach 85% of the rural population.

Education is critical too, particularly with girls in countries where there is a big gender gap as there was in Cambodia in 2000. UNICEF said improving girl's education, particularly at the secondary level, leads to national growth, declining maternity mortality and child mortality rates, with less child stunting. In Cambodia a $41.4 million World Bank project is addressing the shortcomings of education outcomes for half a million students, half of them girls. It was introduced after 2015 when more than 60 % of Cambodian children dropped out of school between 12 and 14. There was a shortage of teachers and morale was low. Thirty new schools were built, teachers training upgraded and over 400 school management committees formed, with community representatives.

Cambodia has continued its battle against HIV/AIDS and in September 2010 the Cambodian Government received a Millenium Development Goal award from the United Nations. The HIV prevalence had dropped to 0.8 percent in 2008 while over 90 percent of HIV positive adults and children were receiving antiretroviral treatment. Over 90 percent of key populations such as sex and entertainment workers, and men having sex with men, had been reached by education campaigns. There had also been nearly a 50 percent decrease in HIV prevalence amongst pregnant women attending antenatal clinics. Of those pregnant women who were HIV positive, over 32 percent received treatment, up from 11.2 percent in 2007.

After a pause during COVID, WHO is hopeful the world will defeat the HIV virus by 2030. It is calling on all countries to reach the 95-95-95 threshold, The three goals are that 95% of all HIV positive individuals are diagnosed, 95% of those diagnosed receive antiretroviral treatment and 95% of those achieve viral suppression. Five countries in Africa have achieved this and another 16 are close. However, almost one quarter 23% of new infections were in Asia and the Pacific.

By 2023 although many goals had been achieved there were still inequalities, with 79% of all new infections in 2022 occurring in men and boys. One in ten HIV positive pregnant women were unable to access prevention services, and the rate of transmission to the newborn was still high at 9.9 %. Just 59 % of children living with HIV were diagnosed and on treatment in 2022.

An estimated 86% of people living with HIV knew their status, with about 11,000 infected people remaining unaware of it. For people with HIV who were diagnosed 99% were on treatment and 98% had achieved viral suppression.

This memoir highlights how difficult it was for the people of Cambodia in 2000 to turn the epidemic around, but with vision, leadership, teamwork, and commitment they did.

The experience for me was extraordinary. It highlighted how little I knew of the world, and my own capacity, and how much larger life is than we generally experience. The epidemic became a personal challenge, and I fought it with everything I had.

I fought it with a great heart, and that is what the country asked of me.

Acknowledgments

The Queensland Writer's Centre for providing me a Flinhart Residency and the opportunity to progress the book.

Laurel Cohn, Editor for her insights during the Next Draft workshops which I have attended several times.

Edwina Shaw for her editorial advice.

The Australian Society of Authors and the Copyright Association for awarding me a mentorship in 2024 and giving me the opportunity to work with ASA Editor Kate Ryan, who has taken me and the manuscript to a higher level.

My beta readers Tricia Adams-Smith, Rae Lindgren and Kath Woodrow for their feedback.

My family, sons Brian and John, their partners Meredith and Linda, and my mother Gill and my sister Liz.

Chapter References

PREFACE

Page 1: A survey found that sixty percent of Cambodian males regularly visited brothels. (Agence France Presse, 199, April 1, *Sex Trade Controls*. South China Morning Post.)

There were already over 5000 AIDS orphans. (Godwin P et.al.(2000) *The HIV/AIDS epidemic in Cambodia. The Contribution of the Health Sector*; Espace, populations, societies, pp 299-308.

Because Fiji and PNG in February 2025 were both facing HIV epidemics, currently the worst in the world after Eastern and Southern Africa. UNAIDS(2024) *Fact Sheet, Global HIV statistics.*

Page 2: Almost 15 years ago, in 2011.. fijivillage.com (1) 0/06/2011) *The threat of HIV/AIDS is like a ticking time bomb for a small island developing State like Fiji*

That didn't happen and now Fiji is facing an HIV outbreak as is PNG. UNAIDS(2024) *Fact Sheet, Global HIV statistics.*

In 2024 alone over 1,093 new cases were recorded UNAIDS, (23 Jan,2025) *As Fiji announces HIV Outbreak UNAIDS echoes calls for a non-discriminatory approach.*

In Papua New Guinea the HIV prevalence rate has reached 1% UNAIDS, (22 Feb 2024,) *UNAIDS regional director urges action to address the HIV epidemic in PNG.*

UNICEF has also urged increasing testing UNICEF, (1 Dec 2024,) *UNICEF sounds alarm on high mother-to-child HIV transmission rates in Papua New Guinea.*

The Solomon Islands too, has seen HIV transmission rise. Tavalulinews.(4, Dec 2024) *ICE drug use a growing concern for HIV transmission.*

By January 2025 two additional cases were suspected, (Ulutah Gina, Solomon Star, (20 Jan, 2025). *Two new HIV unconfirmed cases recorded.*

Dr Jackson Rakei, Director of the Solomon Islands HIV program Tavalulinews. (4, Dec 2024) *ICE drug use a growing concern for HIV transmission.*

In 2015 UNAIDS recognised this risk UNAIDS, (31 March 2015), *Solomon Islands, Global AIDS response progress report 2015.*

CHAPTER ONE ORIENTATION PHNOM PENH

Page 4: Were there rules, invisible to me as a Westerner, or were the drivers visually challenged psychopaths as my Lonely Planet advised? (Taylor, Wheeler, & Robinson, 1996, p. 69, *Cambodia,* Victoria Lonely Planet Publications.

Page 5: American bombs, 500,000 tonnes of them, were dropped between 1969 and 1973 to disrupt the supply route to the Viet Cong. They killed hundreds of thousands of Cambodians and were a major factor in the rise of Pol Pot. (Sophal Ear, 30 November 2023, *Henry Kissinger's bombing campaign likely killed hundreds of thousands of Cambodians- and set path for the ravages of the Khmer Rouge,* Thunderbird School of Global Management, Arizona State University, accessed in the conversation 16th June 2024.)

Cambodia had the highest prevalence rate of amputation in the world, 1 per 236 people. (United Nations Mine Action Service, 2012, *UN in Cambodia Mine Action. UNMAS,* Retrieved from www.unmas.org

The worst year was 1996 when 4,320 people were killed or injured but by 1998 it had dropped to 727. The Ministry of Planning in 1999 estimated there were still 4 to 6 million landmines in the ground. (National Institute of Statistics, Directorate General of Health, Cambodia, June 2001, p 3, *Cambodian demographic and Health Survey 2000.* Retrieved from dhsprogram.com.)

Page 7: The total of those who died during Pol Pot's reign between 1975 and 1979 will never be known; but the Cambodian Genocide Program at Yale University estimates 1.7 million people or one fifth of the population lost their lives (Yale University 2023, *Cambodian Genocide Program.* Retrieved from https:gsp.yale.edu.)

Page 8: The armpit of Cambodia they called it, the border town with Thailand, full of beggars, street kids, and corrupt officials, over 400 km to the Northwest. (Taylor, Wheeler, & Robinson, 1996, p. 69, *Cambodia,* Victoria Lonely Planet Publications.)

CHAPTER TWO POIPET, THE EPICENTRE

Page 10: I was one of 10 expatriates living in a town of around 60,000 people. (1998 census in RC European Commission's Joint Research Centre, 2016. *Sisophon, city in Cambodia.* Retrieved from city.facts.com).

The Lonely Planet 2000 described it as a necessary, but uninteresting town, a service centre for Banteay Meanchey province, and a transport hub (Ray,N. April 2000, *Cambodia 3rd Ed.* Lonely Planet Publications. Australia).

Both roads were awful, and it took over 22 years and $143 million dollars before the road between Sisophon and Battambang was upgraded. (Phnom Pehn Post, 3 December 2021, *Battambang-Sisophon road, National 5, opening in January.*)

The Khmer Rouge and Cambodian troops battled for ascendancy with both sides committing human rights abuses. (Human Rights Watch, 1 March 1995, Cambodia at war. Retrieved from www.refworld.org

The 1999 budget of US$2.4 million for Banteay Meanchey for three years funded farmer training, rural loans, health centres, schools, wells and latrines, literacy programs, roads, irrigation canals and demining activities (UNDP/CARERE2, 1999, *The SEILA Programme Report on Outputs 1 January 1996 -31 March 1999*, Phnom Penh, UNDP/CARERE.)

Page 12: At least they had a good surveillance system supported by the CDC, or Centre for Disease Control and Prevention, but they had yet to tackle the data that emerged (CDC 2014, *CDC in Cambodia* retrieved from www.cdc.gov

Page 17: MSF did provide antiretrovirals in Phnom Penh at Preah Norodom Sihanouk Hospital, but not until July 2001 (United Nations Development Program, 2001, p. 71, *Cambodian Human Development Report, Societal Aspects of the HIV/AIDS epidemic in Cambodia, Progress Report 2001.* Phnom Penh UNDP).

In 2000 antiretrovirals were still very expensive, US $10,000 per patient per year. People paid privately and the treatment was delivered in hospitals under medical supervision. Nowadays, with generic and mass-produced production antiretrovirals cost $63 per person per year (MSF, September 2023, *HIV/AIDS Continuing the fight against a deadly pandemic.* Retrieved from www.msf.org/hiv-dept

Page 18: The Poipet Military Police Commander built the first 49-bedroom hotel, the Neak Meas, for $400,000. There were plans for a casino and twenty thousand people arrived. (Khuy,S.3 April 1998, *Border business poises Poipet for prosperity*, English Cambodia Daily.)

That was appropriate because since their arrival in 1998 they had reduced the sex worker's HIV positive rate from over fifty percent to thirty percent and condom use had increased (Marten, L.2000. *Knowledge, attitudes and practices regarding sexually transmitted diseases in towns of Poipet and Sisophon, Banteay Meanchey*, Phnom Penh MSF).

It was a brutal trade with sixty percent of the sex workers either forced or sold to brothels (United States Department of State,2000, *Country report on Human Rights Practices 2000:Cambodia*, Washington, US Department of State.)

Page 19: Sex was cheap, from $US0.5 to US$1.0, and the average number of clients per night for brothel-based sex workers was four. (Marten, L.2000. *Knowledge, attitudes and practices regarding sexually transmitted diseases in towns of Poipet and Sisophon, Banteay Meanchey*, Phnom Penh MSF).

Page 20: Government workers were paid from US$8 to US$20 per month, and had to resort to private work. (United Nations Development Program, 2001, *Cambodian Human Development Report, Societal Aspects of the HIV/AIDS epidemic in Cambodia, Progress Report 2001*. Phnom Penh UNDP).

Page 21: It was founded in 1997 after the government temporarily closed brothels, then reopened them. (Marten, L.2000, p4, *Knowledge, attitudes and practices regarding sexually transmitted diseases in towns of Poipet and Sisophon, Banteay Meanchey*, Phnom Penh MSF).

There was little chance of success with the court cases though because the traffickers were well connected. (Fordham, G.2003, p 4. *Adolescent and Youth Reproductive Health in Cambodia*. POLICY Project).

Ma Sameat said this further AIDS awareness campaign, combined with the pornography and violence of the sex cafes, led to an increase of rapes with 14-to-15 year old boys raping 10 year old girls. She wanted the sex cafes closed and said she had lobbied the provincial and district heads. Both the Provincial and District Governors denied this.(Shaftel, D. & Ana, P. 5 July 2003, *Economy, The border and vice conspire to make Poipet one of the most dangerous towns in Cambodia*. The Cambodian Daily).

Page 22: During the dry almost one third of rural woman in Cambodia collected water from rivers and streams, lakes, and ponds. (National Institute of Statistics, Directorate General of Health, Cambodia, June 2001, p 19 *Cambodian demographic and Health Survey 2000*. Retrieved from dhsprogram.com.)

Page 24: A survey of 15,000 Khmer women in 2000 showed that 30% of women in Banteay Meanchey farmed their own land and 13% farmed family land. The rest had no land. (National Institute of Statistics, Directorate General of Health, Cambodia, June 2001, pp 224-225, *Cambodian demographic and Health Survey 2000*. Retrieved from dhsprogram.com).

CHAPTER THREE A PROVINCIAL EPIDEMIC.

Page 27: The population in 2000 was around 120,000 people, twice that of Sisophon. (National Institute of Statistics, Directorate General of Health, Cambodia, June 2001, *Cambodian demographic and Health Survey 2000*. Retrieved from dhsprogram.com).

Sexually transmitted infections increased sixfold between September 1992 and January 1993, including HIV. (Buler, M. et al. 2006, *Turning the tide, Cambodia's response to HIV and AIDS 1991-2005.* Phnom Penh:UNAIDS).

In 1997 he included children orphaned by AIDS. United Nations Development Programme, 2001,p 76, *Cambodian Human Development Report, Societal Aspects of the HIV/AIDS epidemic in Cambodia, Progress Report 2001,* Phnom Penh:UNDP)

Cambodia was the first Buddhist country in the world to develop a national Buddhist response to HIV/AIDS. (ESCAP, 2003, p. 117. *HIV/AIDS Prevention, Care and Support: Stories from the community.* UN Retrieved from repository. unescap.org).

Page 28: It was then he founded the Coalition for Peace and Reconciliation and met Maha Ghosananda (Anderson, G. 11 Feb 2008, *Pilgrimages for Peace: Bob Mann on postwar Cambodia.* America. The Jesuit Review (Unclear his surname Maat is incorrect).

Page 29: When Pol Pot's regime collapsed in 1979, only 3000 monks of 60,000 in Cambodia in 1976, were still alive. (Blomfield, S. 28 March 2007, *Maha Ghosanda Obituary,* The Guardian).

Page 33: Before antiretroviral use and the use of Bactrim it killed 75% of people living with AIDS. They caught it when their immunity dropped. Co-trimoxazole or Bactrim was used to prevent it. It was the medication I had recommended to the General and reduced the prevalence of Pneumocystis Pneumonia to around fifty percent.(Centres for Disease Control and Prevention (CDC), October 2004, Vol 10, No 10, *Current Epidemiology of Pneumocystis Pneumonia,* Retrieved wwwnc.cdc.gov>article).

Page 36: This system was ineffective, slow, and dangerous as it detected all metal. Between 1992 and 1998, 200 million pieces of metal were detected, of which just 50,000 or 0.3% were landmines. The workers were at risk of treading on the mines or prodding them too deeply. (MacDonald, J. 2003 Alternatives for landmine Detection, Retrieved from www.rand.org>pubs

Page 35: Following a demining accident in 2022 an official released figures stating between 1997 and 2022 154 deminers had been injured and 31 died. (Sopich, S and Rohany, I, 11 Jan 2022, *Four dead, One injured in Preah Vihear as landmine explodes.* Retrieved from www.camodianess.com

CHAPTER FOUR PLANNING AND NATIONAL SUPPORT

Page 38: I hope we can work together to stop the spread of AIDS, and care for, and show compassion to, those people living with it and their families. Thank you." (Atkin M, Diary Two, April-July, 2000, pp. 14-16).

Page 40: CFDS supported vulnerable families with emergency support, income generation and food security but found it challenging meeting the complex needs of families living with AIDS. (Cambodian Family Development Services,2014, Wiser Directory. Retrieved from www.wiser.directory

Page 41: There was strong legislation and heavy penalties, but because of the high profits and corruption, the legislation was not enforced.(Fordham, G.2003, p 13. *Adolescent and Youth Reproductive Health in Cambodia*. POLICY Project).

Latrines were most uncommon in rural Cambodia in 2000 and most families didn't have them. (National Institute of Statistics, Directorate General of Health, Cambodia, June 2001, p 21., *Cambodian demographic and Health Survey 2000*. Retrieved from dhsprogram.com).

Page 43: Their lives were pleasant, but they were cut off from the rural areas where 84 percent of the population lived. (ESCAP, 2003, p. 116. *HIV/AIDS Prevention, Care and Support: Stories from the community*. UN Retrieved from repository.unescap.org).

It was a huge multi storied building and I was told defence had a large budget. Indeed in 2000 it was US$ 100 million. (macrotrends, *Cambodian Military Spending on defence budget,* Retrieved www.macrotrends)

Page 44: Each program had two government nurses working part time and 3 NGO staff. (United Nations Development Programme, 2001,p 77, *Cambodian Human Development Report, Societal Aspects of the HIV/AIDS epidemic in Cambodia, Progress Report 2001,* Phnom Penh:UNDP).

In Battambang the NGO staff were from KRDA or the Khmer Rural Development Association. (Khmer Rural Development Association,2014, Wiser Directory. Retrieved from www.wiser.directory).

There was a monitoring committee. (United Nations Development Programme, 2001,p 77, *Cambodian Human Development Report, Societal Aspects of the HIV/ AIDS epidemic in Cambodia, Progress Report 2001,* Phnom Penh:UNDP).

Page 45: Two thirds either went to a traditional healers or private clinics and both could be lethal. (National Institute of Statistics, Directorate General of Health, Cambodia, June 2001, pp 34-38, *Cambodian demographic and Health Survey 2000*. Retrieved from dhsprogram.com).

It was suggested health centres and NGOs seek traditional healers and possibly community elders to assist with separating the good practitioners from the harmful ones. (AIDS Technical Working Group, Banteay Meanchey , 2021, p. 9, *Situation Analysis- Banteay Meanchey Province*).

In Banteay Meanchey, almost half, 47% would not refuse sex with their husband if he was HIV positive. (National Institute of Statistics, Directorate General of Health, Cambodia, June 2001, p 222., *Cambodian demographic and Health Survey 2000*. Retrieved from dhsprogram.com).

Page 46: Over half had witnessed AIDS deaths, and births and deaths of sickly children born to infected mothers. (National Institute of Statistics, Directorate General of Health, Cambodia, June 2001, p xxiv., *Cambodian demographic and Health Survey 2000*. Retrieved from dhsprogram.com).

It was uplifting to find faith-based organisations supporting vulnerable villagers. (*Buddhism for Development, Cooperation Committee for Cambodia*, 2004. Retrieved from Buddhism For Development (ccc-cambodia.org)

Around 1000 Thais daily crossed the border to gamble, and in 2001 the Cambodian government collected around $US4 million from the casinos. (Khan, S.2003, *Gambling tourism destroys Cambodia's social fabric*. Koh Santepheap.)

Page 47: Meanwhile the hierarchy profited from both trafficking and the casinos. (Shaftel, D. & Ana, P. 5 July 2003, *Economy, The border and vice conspire to make Poipet one of the most dangerous towns in Cambodia*. The Cambodian Daily).

CHAPTER FIVE A HOLIDAY AND A WORKING HOSPITAL

Page 50: Generally, the country list includes staples such as antibiotics, antimalarials, TB treatments, oral rehydration sachets, analgesics. (Bigdeli, M. Jacobs B. Thomson G, et. al. 28 October 2013, *Access to medicines from a healthy system perspective* , Health Policy Plan pps 692-704).

Page 51: Letter to John, youngest son. Luckily the Quakers have given me some money for two months (Atkin M., Diary Two, April-July, 2000, pp. 146-152).

Page 52: In 2000 the incidence of malaria was almost 81 per 1000 in populations at risk. (WHO, The Global Health Observatory, *Cambodia, Estimated malaria incidence 2000, per 1000 population at risk*. Retrieved from Retrieved from www.who.int>data>gho>)

Page 54: This was Avalokiteshvara, the Buddha of compassion, also found at the Bayon (Ray, N. April 2000, pp 206 and 304, *Cambodia 3ʳᵈ Ed*. Lonely Planet Publications. Australia).

The money was commonly paid from savings (54%) or both interest and non-interest loans (20%). (National Institute of Statistics, Directorate General of Health, Cambodia, June 2001, *Cambodian demographic and Health Survey 2000.* Retrieved from dhsprogram.com.)

The Health Equity fund introduced in 2016 addressed the problem by providing free access to the poorest people for 2.6 million outpatient visits and 190,000 hospital visits annually. (World Bank, 21 April 2019, Cambodia: Reducing poverty and sharing prosperity. Retrieved from www.worldbank.org).

Page 55: When the villagers returned to farming, they became vulnerable, and the reservoir became a protected area in 1999. (Rouen, V. 2 August 2001, Authorities move to protect endangered cranes. Retrieved from english. cambodiandaily.com.).

Page 58: Many families disappeared, but 80 shifted onto land that had not been demined and one person lost a leg. Even the Governor seemed embarrassed by it. (Lor, C. 3 July 2000 pp 1-2) *Poipet Evictions, Arrests of Protestors decried,* The Cambodian Daily.

CHAPTER SIX AIDS ZOO AND ANOTHER EPICENTRE BOEUNG TRAKOUN

Page 60: The monks were provided with basic training about HIV/AIDS so they could provide education, care, and support in their communities (UNESCAP, 2003. *HIV/AIDS Prevention, Care and Support: Stories from the community.* Retrieved from repository.unescap.org).

Page 61: While the man could choose who he married the woman could not. (Heuveline. P. & Nakphong, M. 2023, *Contemporary marriage in Cambodia.* Journal of family issues.)

Page 61: Half of Cambodian women were married by 20, and this had been the case for two decades. Eighty five percent were married by 25. (National Institute of Statistics, Directorate General of Health, Cambodia, June 2001, pp 97-98, *Cambodian demographic and Health Survey 2000.* Retrieved from dhsprogram.com).

They were higher when the women were over 25 when they married, when the man was unemployed or if the woman had a much higher educational status. (Heuveline. P. & Nakphong, M. 2023, *Contemporary marriage in Cambodia.* Journal of family issues.)

The survey of 15,000 women in 2000 bore this out with less than 1% of married women using them. (National Institute of Statistics, Directorate

General of Health, Cambodia, June 2001, pp 79-81, *Cambodian demographic and Health Survey 2000*. Retrieved from dhsprogram.com).

Page 62: These figures were based on the East West Centre's Asian Epidemic Model.(Sisowath, D.C. 2006, pp 53-75, *Cambodia fighting a rising tide. The response to AIDS in East Asia, Tokyo,* Japan Centre for International Exchange.)

Page 66: Many were illiterate, lacked numeracy skills and remained in permanent debt to the brothel owner. (Marten, L.2000. p 24, p 33, *Knowledge, attitudes and practices regarding sexually transmitted diseases in towns of Poipet and Sisophon, Banteay Meanchey,* Phnom Penh MSF).

The brothel owner was shocked when I told her around one third to one half of these border sex workers had HIV. (Godwin P et.al. (2000) pp 299-308.*The HIV/AIDS epidemic in Cambodia: The Contribution of the Health Sector,* Retrieved Espace,populations,societies,).

Page 67: They would do more survey work of the high-risk groups and areas over the following month and their findings would also be presented to the District Health Director. (Atkin M., *Diary Three, July-September, 2000,* pp. 64, 66-80).

CHAPTER SEVEN BROTHELS AND THE HUNDRED PERCENT CONDOM PROGRAM.

Page 69: Maternity related deaths were one of the leading causes of death for women between 15 and 49 years. In 2000, around 430 women out of 100,000 who gave birth, died. Most deaths were preventable. (Mallick, L., Allen, C. Hong, R.. Jan 2018, *fig 2, p2, Maternal Mortality Rate, Cambodia 2000, 2005, 2010,2014* Cambodian Demographic and Health Surveys) Trends in Maternal and Child Health in Cambodia 2000-2014), USAID.)

Page 69: By comparison in Australia, between 2000 and 2002 the maternal mortality rate was 11.1 per 100,000 women. (Australian Institute of Health and Welfare, 2006, Table 5, p 9, *Maternal deaths in Australia 2000-2002.*)

Two thirds of grandparents supported their orphaned grandchildren and half of these did so, despite financial hardship. (Orbach, D., *Committed to caring, Older women and HIV/AIDS in Cambodia, Thailand and Vietnam,* Help Age International).

Page 71: Paragraph beginning, there wasn't enough money in villages to generate funds for self-help groups, but from 2003 to 2007 Family Health International supported older carers and People living with AIDS (PLWHA) in 19 villages in Battambang. (Orbach, D., *Committed to caring, Older women and HIV/AIDS in Cambodia, Thailand and Vietnam,* Help Age International).

Paragraph beginning,' late in August I was back in Battambang talking with the military and ending with, 'the rate of condom use with sex workers amongst the military rose by 16% to 81% in 2001. (ESCAP, 2003, pp 19-21. *HIV/AIDS Prevention, Care and Support: Stories from the community.* UN Retrieved from repository.unescap.org).

This Regional Military Hospital (Region 5) received support from June 2004 from the Ministry of National Defence, NCHADS and FHI.(Tap, W.S. 2005, p 60, *Mapping Cambodia's response to HIV/AIDS*, Phnom Penh, NCHADS).

Page 75: The Vice Governor was head of the Condom Monitoring and Evaluation Committee. (World Bank, 21 April, 2004, *Document of the World Bank Project Performance and Assessment Report No 28648.* Retrieved from www. worldbank.org).

Page 75: Paragraph beginning, 'a MSF worker from Phnom Penh supported the Cambodian Prostitutes Union. It was founded by Tia, a 28-year-old woman, forced into prostitution after she fled an abusive relationship. (Boyce, D. 17 June 1999, *Together sex workers speak with a louder voice.* Retrieved from feministarchives.isiswomen.org).

Page 76: Their union survived. (Union Aid Abroad, 13 November 2017, *Working for rights and dignity of sex workers in Cambodia.* Retrieved from www. apheda.org.au).

CHAPTER EIGHT PAILIN AND THE KHMER ROUGE

Page 79: Paragraph from, 'there were drunken men driving a tractor up and down the road', and ending,'this dropped to 12 percent for women with secondary or higher education.' (National Institute of Statistics, Directorate General of Health, Cambodia, June 2001, *Cambodian demographic and Health Survey 2000.* Retrieved from dhsprogram.com). HSS

Page 79-80: In 1999 the HIV Surveillance Study (HSS) showed from 10 to 25% of the brothel-based sex workers were HIV positive. The virus was also crossing into the general population. The prevalence in antenatal women below 30 was 2.3%, while antenatal women above 30 had a rate of 4.5%. (Ministry of Health Cambodia, NCHADS, 2000, *Sentinel Surveillance Study, HSS Results 1999*, p 39., Retrieved from www.nchads.org).

Page 80: Their clients were at risk from sepsis and tetanus, and sometimes died. (National Institute of Statistics, Directorate General of Health, Cambodia, June 2001, pp. 71-72, *Cambodian demographic and Health Survey 2000.* Retrieved from dhsprogram.com).

Sex workers were also at risk with one quarter having at least one abortion, while less than 5 percent using contraception. (Delvaux, T., Seng, S., Laga, M., May 2023, *The need for family planning and safe abortion services among women sex workers seeking STI care in Cambodia*. Retrieved from pubmed.ncbi. nim.nih.gov).

The stupa was erected in the honour of Yiey Yat Yat, a sorceress who warned the Kola to stop killing her animals. She said when they stopped hunting, they would be rewarded. They went into the jungle and saw an otter playing near a stream and when the otter opened his mouth, it was full of jewels. The jewels were still there and when it rained heavily the villagers came to look for them, as they washed down the gravel road. (Zepp, R. (2000 May, *Pailin: Town of miners and deminers*. Retrieved andybrouwer.co.uk).

Page 82: The deadly plasmodium falciparum had become resistant, not only to Artemisinin but to its partner drug Piperaquine (Roberts, L., 21 April 2016, *Drug resistance triggers war to wipe out malaria in the Mekong Region*. Retrieved from science.org).

This dropped the incidence of malaria in the population in that area from 77.8 per 1000 in 2000 to 5.8 per 1000 in 2020. (Asian Development Bank, 2023, *Greater Mekong Subregion Border Areas Health Project, RRP CAM 53290*. Retrieved from adb.org 53290).

Page 83: In 2000 the Lonely Planet said there was little point going to Pailin unless you liked hanging out with geriatrics responsible for mass murder. (Ray, N., April 2000,p 205, *Cambodia 3rd Edition*, Lonely Planet Publications, Australia).

In the recent edition they spoke of the two wats and a pleasant waterfall. (Ray, N, Dailly,M. & Eimer, D. p 168 *Lonely Planet Cambodia* , 2023, Lonely Planet Publications, Australia).

Pailin has grown. In 2000 there were 3000 people in Pailin town and 8000 people in the province. In 2023 there were almost ten times that number; 79,000 people in the province. (cityfacts, 2015, *Pailin*. Retrieved from city-facts.com).

Page 84: We are getting together a proposal for the other difficult border district Thma Puok which includes Boeun Trakoun and it is likely to get money next year.. (Atkin M., *Diary Five, October- January, 2000-2001*, p. 6).

There were rags strung around it and men banging drums and shouting sporadically at the circling birds. (Atkin M., *Diary Five, October- January, 2000-2001*, p.7).

Page 84 to 85: Begins, 'It's been a while since I wrote,' and ends.'I hear Dad's doing a locum in Coff's Harbour. How I long to see them again.' (Atkin M., *Diary Five,October- January, 2000-2001*, pp. 23-27).

CHAPTER NINE A FAMILY TRAGEDY, TOURING, CHRISTMAS

Page 86: The damage caused to infrastructure and crops reached $US 50 million (Asian Disaster Reduction Centre, 26 July 2000, Cambodia: Flood: 2000/08. Retrieved from www.adrc.asia).

Page 88: At least it was a break from middle aged European men and young Khmer girls. (Atkin M., *Diary Five,October- January, 2000-2001*, pp. 48-50).

Page 89: China agreed to give Cambodia $US12 million in grant aid and loans and offered help to flood victims (Agence France-Press, 14 November 2000, *Visit to Cambodia by China's leader.* Retrieved from nytimes.com).

There are also old colonial houses some abandoned. (Atkin M., *Diary Five,October- January, 2000-2001*, pp. 55-66).

Page 90: Paragraph beginning, 'the French colonialists built it in 1925, or more accurately, it was built by indentured Khmer labourers 1000 of whom lost their lives.' Up to, 'in 1972 the hill station was abandoned for the second time.' (Kuriositas, 21 December 2021, *Bokor Hill Station, Cambodia's abandoned town*, Retrieved kuriositas.com.).

Page 91: They supported them during the eighties with military training, preferring them to the Soviet backed Vietnamese and denied the genocide taking place during Pol Pot's era. (Harper, T.H., 13 Feb 2023, *Cambodia's triumph and tragedy: The UN's greatest experiment 30 years on.* Retrieved from hir.harvard.edu.)

The Chinese plan to swamp the site with luxury houses, a casino, a hotel, and a luxury go kart track. (Froelich,P, 22 February 2022, *How China is destroying a precious Cambodian paradise.* Retrieved from nypost.).

CHAPTER TEN WORKING WITH NGOS AND THE SITUATION ANALYSIS

Page 95: HALO also employed men and women from the communities they worked in, boosting local economies (HALO, 13 December 2016, *25 years making their communities safer, HALO Cambodia*, Retrieved from halotrust.org.).

Page 96: They did excellent work and were the one of two Cambodian NGOs included in a regional UN report featuring HIV/AIDS initiatives. (ESCAP,

2003, p. 117. *HIV/AIDS Prevention, Care and Support: Stories from the community.* UN Retrieved from repository.unescap.org).

Page 97: Not only patients, but nurses and doctors felt the situation was hopeless. *(AIDS Technical Working Group Banteay Meanchey , 2001 , p. 5).*

Page 100: Sadly, he was leaving Battambang in February, but I asked if he could come back every three months to help with proposals. (Atkin M , *Diary Six, January-April, 2001,* p. 13).

Only 10 percent of women in Banteay Meanchey had heard about the law against sexual trafficking while it was over one half nationally. (National Institute of Statistics, Directorate General of Health, Cambodia, June 2001,pp 228-229, *Cambodian demographic and Health Survey 2000.* Retrieved from dhsprogram.com.)

CHAPTER ELEVEN CHINESE NEW YEAR 2001

Page 102: In 2002 Cambodia had one of the highest TB prevalence rates in the world with more than 1500 cases per 100,000 people (WHO, 1 October 2012, *Cambodia turns a TB health crisis into an opportunity.* Retrieved from who.int.).

By comparison Australia in 2001 had 5.1 cases per 100,000 people (Department of Health and Aged Care, Australia, 18 December 2002, *Tuberculosis Notifications in Australia 2001,* Retrieved from www1.health.gov. au/internet/main/).

In 2001 a survey found that 64% of Cambodians were infected with the TB bacteria but not all had symptoms. (Eang,M., Chheng, P., Natpratan, C., & Kimmerling, M., May 2007, Lessons from TB/HIV integration in Cambodia. Retrieved from ncbi.nih.gov.).

In 2002 almost one quarter of the population or 23.6% was malnourished. By 2021 that had dropped to 6%. (Knoema,2022. Cambodian Food Security Prevalence of undernourishment as share of the population. Retrieved from knoema.com).

HIV prevalence among TB patients increased from 2.5% in 1995 to 10% in 2005. (Eang,M., Chheng, P., Natpratan, C., & Kimmerling, M., May 2007, *Lessons from TB/HIV integration in Cambodia.* Retrieved from ncbi.nih.gov.).

Page 103: A recent study confirms there is an association between the exposure of fathers to pesticides and the higher incidence of cleft palates in their children (Suhi,J., Romitti,P., & et. al., 27 March 2020, *Parental occupational pesticide exposure and nonsyndromic orofacial clefts.* Retrieved from ncbi.nim.nih.gov.).

A survey in 2000 of 15,000 women showed that in Cambodia one in ten children died before their first birthday with major childhood illnesses including diarrhoea, fever and respiratory infections. (National Institute of Statistics, Directorate General of Health, Cambodia, June 2001, pp 121-125, Cambodian demographic and Health Survey 2000. Retrieved from dhsprogram.com.)

In Banteay Meanchey 20 % of children under five had diarrhoea in the previous fortnight. (National Institute of Statistics, Directorate General of Health, Cambodia, June 2001, pp 121-125, Cambodian demographic and Health Survey 2000. Retrieved from dhsprogram.com.)

Page 103: During the dry almost one third of rural woman in Cambodia had to get water from rivers and streams, lakes, and ponds. (National Institute of Statistics, Directorate General of Health, Cambodia, June 2001,p 19, *Cambodian demographic and Health Survey 2000*. Retrieved from dhsprogram.com.)

Page 104: PSI was established in Cambodia in 1993 and launched a social market condom for Number One Condoms which are still widely used. They have provided over 9 million condoms. (PSI, September 2023, Retrieved from psi.org.kh. subtitled who we are.).

Page 105: A survey from 2000 showed that Khmer women usually married at 20, with almost 90% virgins at the time of marriage. (National Institute of Statistics, Directorate General of Health, Cambodia, June 2001, *Cambodian demographic and Health Survey 2000*.pp 97-98, Retrieved from dhsprogram.com.).

Page 106: In the end it took RAMSI, the Regional Assistance Mission to Solomon Islands, and 3 billion dollars. (Dobell, G., 10 April 2017, *Saving Solomon Islands from crocodiles: 14 years of RAMSI*, Retrieved from www. aspistrategist.org.au.)

Page 107: Once they corrected these problems their yields increased, and they used less seed. The rice straw which the cows fed on was left in the fields to increase fertility. (Winarto, Y.T., 2004, *Farmer field school, farmer life school and farmer's club for enriching knowledge and empowering farmers: A case study in Cambodia* Retrieved from semanticscholar.org.)

CHAPTER TWELVE SIEM REAP

Page 111: A more recent theory suggests inhabitants left after climate change caused a major drought. (University of Sydney, 14 April 2020, *Climate change and the collapse of Angkor Wat*, Retrieved from www.sydney.edu.au>news).

It was as though the evil this country had endured and would endure could be vanquished by that face. (Atkin M. *Diary Six, January-April, 2001,* pp. 129-130).

Page 111: His second wife, the elder sister of his first who had died, was Rajendradevi, a renowned poet, philosopher, and scientist. (Cambodian Museum, 2023, *Jayavarman VII,* Retrieved from cambodia.museum.info).

Khmer society, over one thousand years ago, was well ahead of the West, when almost the only woman celebrated was the Virgin Mary (Atkin M. *Diary Six, January-April, 2001,* pp. 132-134).

It was the only temple not built by a King but by a counsellor to a King Jayavarman V. He was a Brahmin, a priest and doctor, also of royal descent. He began building the temple in 967 (tourism cambodia, 2023, *Banteay Srei-Siem Reap,* Retrieved from tourismcambodia.com).

Page 112: I glimpsed myself in some nearby mirror and my face had changed. I was young again. (Atkin M. *Diary Six, January-April, 2001,* p. 134).

Page 113: The vaccination coverage then was 45%. (National Institute of Statistics, Directorate General of Health, Cambodia, June 2001, *Cambodian demographic and Health Survey 2000.* Retrieved from dhsprogram.com.).

CHAPTER THIRTEEN MALAI AND THE KHMER ROUGE

Page 117: They returned to their districts in the rainy season to plant, grow and harvest their rice. We discussed how this was another way the virus could spread. (Atkin M. , *Diary Six, January-April, 2001,* pp. 183-185).

Page 118: Anti-trafficking laws were passed in June 2008 and the police vigorously enforced them (Chrann,C. 28 October 2008, *Police rescue women from torture, forced sex in B'bang brothel,* Retrieved from phnompenhpost.com).

They were armed with AK47s and machetes and as the husband of the female Commander, also a Commander observed soberly, knew how to use them. (Fitzgerald, T. 2 May 1997, *KR women lay down law to brothels.* Retrieved from phnompenhpost.com).

Page 118: There were thatched huts, some with clay kilns out the back. It was a productive visit and I enjoyed it. (Atkin M. *Diary Six, January-April, 2001,* pp. 190-191).

Page 119: The fifty thousand people who lived in the district in 2022 were now more affluent (Sivutha, N. 14 June 2022, *Malai district; From minefields to plantations.* Retrieved from phnompenh.post.com).

Page 120: Women here got married at 20 and had 4 children. (National

Institute of Statistics, Directorate General of Health, Cambodia, June 2001, *Cambodian demographic and Health Survey 2000*.pp 97-98, Retrieved from dhsprogram.com.)

During that time is estimated at least 1.7 million people or one fifth of the population lost their lives. (Yale University 2023, *Cambodian Genocide Program*. Retrieved from https:gsp.yale.edu.)

On March 14 1992 the United Nations Transitional Authority in Cambodia ruled for 18 months in an attempt to stabilise the country so democracy could be established. (Harper, T.H., 13 Feb 2023, *Cambodia's triumph and tragedy: The UN's greatest experiment 30 years on*. Retrieved from hir.harvard.edu.)

Page 121: At that stage US suspended all non-humanitarian aid to Cambodia. Thirty thousand Cambodians fled to Thailand to escape the fighting. The US embassy however did not provide asylum to Cambodians facing political persecution.(UNHCR, Human Rights Watch, 1 August 1997, *Cambodia: Aftermath of the Coup*, Retrieved from refworld.org).

Garment exports accounted for 77 percent of Cambodia's total exports in 2000 and earnt $US 985 million. The garment exports continued growing until 2004 when quotas were established.(Bargawi, O. October 2005, *Cambodia's Garment Industry- Origins and future prospects*. Economic and Statistics Analysis Unit, Overseas Development Institute London, Retrieved from https://ideas.repec.org).

They were on their way to Banteay Meanchey. I had been in Cambodia almost a year and this was the best gift we could be given. (Atkin M. *Diary Six, January-April*, 2001, p. 226).

Page 121: I had to keep my mobile on, which I had avoided most of my life. I always preferred to work on one thing at a time. (Atkin M. *Diary Seven, April-July*, 2001, p. 227).

Page 122: He had been in a very difficult situation and was helped by a South Malaitan relative. (Atkin M., *Diary Six, January-April*, 2001, pp. 254-266).

Page 123: When the rain stopped, I walked back and found some white flowers with an exquisite smell in my garden. (Atkin M. *Diary Six, January-April*, 2001, p. 228).

CHAPTER FOURTEEN DONORS RETURN

Page 124: They trained peer educators and supported thousands of garment workers with information about sexual reproductive and maternal health. (Care,25 November 2014, *Bipartisan Congressional Delegation travels with CARE to see better solution to women's health in Cambodia.* Retrieved from www.care. org).

Your willingness to discuss important health issues in the Cambodian context has helped USAID Cambodia's Office of Public Health to assess its current portfolio and start to develop a new long-term strategy given the realities of the current health situation in Cambodia. (Connolly, Letter of thanks to Margaret Atkin HIV/AIDS Coordinator Banteay Meanchey Province UNDP , 2001)

By October 2001 they had released their strategy for Cambodia for 2002 to 2005. It led to the establishment of three clinics in Banteay Meanchey and more support for KHANA.(USAID, October 2001, *USAID/Cambodia Interim PHN Strategy 2002-2005.* Retrieved from usaid.gov).

Page 125: KHANA (Khmer HIV/AIDS NGO Alliance) is an NGO which in 2003 provided support to over 40 NGOs working in the HIV/AIDS and STI field. (ESCAP, 2003, p. 117. *HIV/AIDS Prevention, Care and Support: Stories from the community.* UN Retrieved from repository.unescap.org).

Page 125: If they did, the clinic tested for trichomoniasis and syphilis, but not chlamydia or gonorrhoea (World Bank , 21 April 2004, *Document of the World Bank Project Performance and Assessment Report No 28648,* p. 13). Retrieved from www.worldbank.org).

Page 125: Untreated chlamydia and gonorrhoea could lead to inflammatory pelvic disease and infertility (Better Health , 2023, *Chlamydia.* Retrieved from betterhealth.vic.gov.au).

Presumptive treatment could be used in the short-term but was not a long-term solution (Steen, R. & Dallabetta, G., November 2003, *Sexually transmitted infection control with sex workers.* Retrieved from jstor.org.)

The results were lower than in 1996, but the same as a similar study in 2001. (Sopheap, H., Morineau, G. & Neal, J., 12 December 2008, *Sustained high prevalence of sexually transmitted infections among female sex workers in Cambodia.* Retrieved from bmcinfectdis.biomedcentral.com.)

Page 126: They worked at border crossings to monitor and support women and children encountering trafficking and violence and were considering working there. (CWCC, 4 November 2023, *SMART project.* Retrieved from www.cwcc.org.kh).

Page 126: A couple of weeks earlier, I had contacted Cambodian Family Development Services, an international NGO based at Tuol Pongro. They supported income generation, food security and provided counselling.

(Cambodian Women's Crisis Centre, 2014, Wiser Directory. Retrieved from www.wiser.directory).

Page 129: Roasting for three days to a month improved overall health after birth and abortions. A survey of 15,000 women in 2000 stated that almost 90% of Khmer women practised roasting for at least three days after birth, including over sixty percent of educated women. (National Institute of Statistics, Directorate General of Health, Cambodia, June 2001, pp 144-146, *Cambodian demographic and Health Survey 2000*. Retrieved from dhsprogram.com.)

CHAPTER FIFTEEN TURNING THE TIDE – OVERLOOKED BORDER TROOPS

Page 133: Arlys knew of 150 orphans in the Mongol Borei District, just one of seven districts in Banteay Meanchey Province. It was estimated there were 55,000 nationwide. (ESCAP, 2003, *HIV/AIDS Prevention, Care and Support: Stories from the community*. UN Retrieved from repository.unescap.org).

The survey found more than half of all Cambodian children had experienced physical violence before 18, and a quarter emotional abuse. Around 5% had been sexually abused. (Ministry of Women's Affairs, UNICEF Cambodia, US Centers for Disease Control and Prevention. *Findings from Cambodia's Violence Against Children Survey 2013*. P. 20. Cambodia: Ministry of Women's Affairs, 2014.)

Page 134: That was the aim of the Commune Committees formed in 2004 for women and children (CCWCs). They reported to officials in the Ministry of Social Affairs/Veterans and Youth. (Jordanwood, M, 2016, *Role of commune committees for women and children and informal community-based child protection mechanisms in Cambodia*. Retrieved from wvi.org).

In 2002 the rate of transmission from husbands to wives was 42%, and the most common way HIV was spread. (National AIDS Authority, NAA, April 2003, *Cambodian Report on follow-up to the Declaration of Commitment on HIV/ AIDS (UNGASS)*. Phnom Penh: UNAIDS).

Nationally a third of married woman didn't believe they could refuse sex if their husbands were HIV positive. (National Institute of Statistics, Directorate General of Health, Cambodia, June 2001, p 221, *Cambodian demographic and Health Survey 2000*. Retrieved from dhsprogram.com.)

Page 134: Less than 1% of married couples used condoms because as Sopheak told me condoms were associated with brothels. (National Institute of Statistics, Directorate General of Health, Cambodia, June 2001, pps. 79-81, *Cambodian demographic and Health Survey 2000*. Retrieved from dhsprogram.com.)

The rate of maternal to child transmission was the second highest rate of transmission at 2.8%. Transmission could be stopped with antiretroviral treatment but in 2002 there were 4,536 HIV positive pregnant women and just over 2% had access to antiretrovirals. (National AIDS Authority, NAA, April 2003, *Cambodian Report on follow-up to the Declaration of Commitment on HIV/AIDS (UNGASS)*. Phnom Penh: UNAIDS).

Page 135: Since 2013 UNFPA have supported the Ministry of Education Youth and Sport with the Life Skills Education Program in 25% of the upper primary and secondary schools in the country and this has now been expanded. (United Nations Population Fund Cambodia ,18/01/2016, *Education for a Healthy Future: Integrating Comprehensive Sexuality Education into the School Curriculum* Retrieved from http://cambodia.unfpa.org.)

Page 137: The report suggested, messaging and condoms be available in commercial sex establishments and men be encouraged to have sex prior to engaging in heavy drinking. (Smith, R., December 2008, *Lets go for a walk, Sexual decision making among clients of female entertainment workers in Phnom Penh*, Washington: PSI).

Page 138: By 2002 70% of the military in Cambodia had peer educator programs and condoms, together with 25% of the police. (National AIDS Authority, NAA, April 2003, *Cambodian Report on follow-up to the Declaration of Commitment on HIV/AIDS (UNGASS)*. Phnom Penh: UNAIDS).

The project provided roads, tracks to rural plots, infrastructure for water supply, and accessible schools and health clinics (World Bank, 29 October 2019, *Cambodia: Reducing Poverty and sharing Prosperity,* Retrieved from worldbank.org).

Page 139: Almost forty percent of the patients who needed medication were receiving it. (Charles, M., 2006, *HIV epidemic in Cambodia, one of the poorest countries in Southeast Asia, a success story.* Retrieved from ncbi.nim.nih.gov.)

Page 140: Otherwise, the groups that were still at risk could reinfect the others. (Charles, M., 2006, *HIV epidemic in Cambodia, one of the poorest countries in Southeast Asia, a success story.* Retrieved from ncbi.nim.nih.gov.)

Page 141: Marie Stopes in their Cambodian website in 2023 advertised Marie Stopes ladies, midwives and doctors were able to provide services in rural areas. (Marie Stopes, 2023, *Marie Stopes Ladies*. Retrieved from mariestopes.org.kh)

Page 141: Another pro-choice organisation, MSI, mentions self -managed abortion for pregnancies up to three months. (MSI Asia Pacific, 28 September 2020, Self-managed abortions in Cambodia, Retrieved from www.msichoices. org.au).

In our situation analysis we acknowledged the problem and suggested a women's clinic be provided. (AIDS Technical Working Group Banteay Meanchey, 2001, p.13).

Homosexuality was not widely discussed in Cambodia at that time and young men were often unaware of it (AIDS Technical Working Group, Banteay Meanchey, 2021, p.19).

It was a vulnerable group. An FHI report from 2000 in Phnom Penh identified that of the men who had sex with men surveyed, 26% had an STI and 14% were HIV positive. (National AIDS Authority, NAA, April 2003, *Cambodian Report on follow-up to the Declaration of Commitment on HIV/AIDS (UNGASS).* Phnom Penh: UNAIDS).

If they like you, they tell you. Life is too short and too precious to lie or pretend. (Atkin M., *Diary Seven, April-July, 2001*, p. 126).

CHAPTER SIXTEEN MARGINALIZED WOMEN AND CHILDREN

Page 142: As the situation analysis pointed out, there were no national guidelines for providing symptomatic level A treatment to mobile patients, including those with diarrhoea, skin problems and pain (*AIDS Technical Working Group, Banteay Meanchey, 2021,* p. 4).

Page 145: The national survey of 15,000 women in 2000 showed the depth of the gender gap in Banteay Meanchey, one of the least developed provinces.

This was not only in relation to men, but women from other provinces. While half of the women in Banteay Meanchey couldn't read, over 90 percent of women in Phnom Penh could. (National Institute of Statistics, Directorate General of Health, Cambodia, June 2001, *Cambodian demographic and Health Survey 2000,* p.45-46, Retrieved from dhsprogram.com.)

More than a third of women in Banteay Meanchey hadn't been to school and half believed it was more important to educate boys than girls. (National Institute of Statistics, Directorate General of Health, Cambodia, June 2001, *Cambodian demographic and Health Survey 2000.* Pp 45-46 and p 217, Retrieved from dhsprogram.com.)

More than half of the women in Banteay Meanchey believed a woman shouldn't work outside the home and the family rice-fields. (National Institute of Statistics, Directorate General of Health, Cambodia, June 2001, pp 47-49, *Cambodian demographic and Health Survey 2000.* Retrieved from dhsprogram.com.)

Almost 90 percent of the Banteay Meanchey women had no knowledge of their legal rights in relation to in relation to marriage, violence and labour, yet 1 in 6 women throughout Cambodia experienced sexual violence. (National Institute of Statistics, Directorate General of Health, Cambodia, June 2001, pp 228-229 and pp 233-240, *Cambodian demographic and Health Survey 2000.* Retrieved from dhsprogram.com.)

Page 146: It was suggested gender issues be included in the school curriculum. (AIDS Technical Working Group, Banteay Meanchey, 2021, p. 16)

Page 146: Nationally, other considerations included limiting youth access to alcohol, strengthened law enforcement and responsible service delivery. (Yeung, W., Leong, W., Khoun,K., et. al., September 2015, *Alcohol use disorder and heavy episodic drinking in rural communities in Cambodia.* Retrieved from resarchgate.net.)

Page 148: By 2003 they provided support for 35 people living with HIV/AIDS and 133 children affected by AIDS. (ESCAP, 2003, p. 89. *HIV/AIDS Prevention, Care and Support: Stories from the community.* UN Retrieved from repository. unescap.org).

Page 148: Her 18-year-old daughter then returned to live with them. (ESCAP, 2003, p. 89. *HIV/AIDS Prevention, Care and Support: Stories from the community.* UN Retrieved from repository.unescap.org).

Page 149: We advocated a youth advisor be employed to work with working groups, the department of Education, increase skills in service providers and carry out research (AIDS Technical Working Group, Banteay Meanchey, 2021, p. 12).

Page 149: He advocated a policy be designed, research be carried out, NGOs participate in interagency working groups, suitable visual media be developed and the capacity of public servants in ministries be developed. (Fordham, G., 2003, *Adolescent and Youth Reproductive Health in Cambodia.* POLICY Project).

Page 150: Paragraph beginning, 'it was estimated in a survey carried out in Phnom Penh that injection of drugs had increased from 0.6% of all drug use in 2000 to 10% in 2004' and ending in, 'Risks included 40 % of the injecting drug users having multiple sex partners and rarely using condoms, while 47% sold blood and shared needles. (Eang,M., Chheng, P., Natpratan, C., & Kimmerling, M., May 2007, *Lessons from TB/HIV integration in Cambodia.* Retrieved from ncbi.nih.gov.).

In Banteay Meanchey there were two, one run by the Military Police and another by the Ministry of Social Affairs, Veterans, and Youth Rehabilitation. (Brigadier General Thong Sokunthea & Dr Chhit Sophal, 2010, *Cambodia, Drug*

Abuse and Drug Dependence Treatment Situation 2008. Retrieved from www. unodc.org).

It was conducted by the International Network of Treatment and Rehabilitation Centres (Treatnet). Follow up workshops were held. (UNODC, 24 November 2010, *Cambodia hosts community-based drug dependence treatment workshop.* Retrieved from unodc.org).

CHAPTER SEVENTEEN BOUENG TRAKOUN TRANSFORMED & DEPARTURE

Page 153: I finally arrived at 4pm and discovered a huge electricity bill, US$70 for the month, and I wasn't there. (Atkin M., *Diary Seven, April-July, 2001,* pp. 219-220).

The Cambodian Red Cross (CRC) would work with Police and finally the Social Environment Agricultural Development Organisation (SEADO) and CRC would do more work with schools (Atkin M., *Diary Seven, April-July, 2001,* pp. 219-220).

Page 154: We had learnt from this pilot project and hoped similar projects could be run in other districts (Atkin M., *Diary Seven, April-July, 2001,* pp. 236, 332-333).

Page 154 -155: Haemorrhage during and after childbirth was one of the three major reasons why the maternal mortality rate in Cambodia was so high, 437 maternal deaths per 100,000 live births. The other two causes were eclampsia and deaths following abortions. (Mallick, L., Allen, C. Hong, R.. Jan 2018, fig 2, p2, Maternal Mortality Rate, Cambodia 2000, 2005, 2010,2014 Cambodian Demographic and Health Surveys) Trends in Maternal and Child Health in Cambodia 2000-2014), USAID.)

Page 157: Paragraph from, 'it wasn't until December 2005 they got what they needed. It was then the US Ambassador opened an HIV/AIDS testing and treatment clinic,' and ending in, besides an HIV in-patient unit, health staff were trained, laboratory equipment and reagents provided, an isolation unit built for AIDS patients with TB, an X Ray machine provided, meals provided to patients, and the maternity wing upgraded. (US Embassy Cambodia 10 May 2007, *Fighting HIV/AIDS in Banteay Meanchey Province, Poipet Health Centre.* Retrieved from kh.usembassy.gov).

Page 158: Over 100 people died, and houses, roads and wells were destroyed. (Asian Disaster Reduction Centre, 26 July, 21 and 29 September 2000, Cambodia Flood:2000/08. Retrieved from www.adrc.asia.)

POSTSCRIPT

Page 163: Unlike the Solomons I have little desire to return to Cambodia, although in 2023, 5.45 million other tourists visited Cambodia and perhaps that's why. (Xinhua Net, 22 March 2024, *Cambodia records nearly 1mln in'l tourists in January February period*, Retrieved https//english.news.cn).

Page 163: Whereas 40 % of the population was under the poverty line in 2009 this dropped by more than half to 18% in 2020. (New Straits Times, 2 August, 2022, *Cambodia's poverty rate drops by over 22 % in last ten years* Retrieved from https://www.nst.com.my/world/region/2022/08/818659/cambodias-poverty-rate-drops-over-22-cent-last-ten-years.).

The World Bank said this was because of stability and good economic management, with Cambodian workers moving from agriculture to manufacturing and services, with urban areas growing. (World Bank Group, 28 November 2022, *Cambodia Poverty Assessment 2022: Toward a more inclusive and resilient Cambodia,* Retrieved from www.worldbank.org/en/country/cambodia/publication/cambodia-poverty-assessment-2022-toward-a-more-inclusive-and-resilient-cambodia).

In 2022, GDP per capita for Cambodia was US 1760 dollars, up from 364 dollars in 2003.(Knoema, 2023, Cambodia, National Accounts Gross Domestic Product, Retrieved https://knoema.com/atlas/Cambodia/topics/Economy/National-Accounts-Gross-Domestic-Product/GDP-per-capita)

The average world GDP per capita was US$12,600 in 2022. (World Bank Retrieved https://data.worldbank.org/indicator/NY.GDP.PCAP.CD?).

Average life expectancy increased from 59 in 2000 to 71.5 in 2024.(World Bank 2024, Retrieved www.data.worldbank.org/indicator/SP.DYN.LE00.IN?locations=K

There were just 350 villages without power in early 2022. (UNDP Cambodia, 20 March 2022 *Reaching Cambodia's last mile with inclusive and sustainable energy access,* Retrieved from https://www.undp.org/cambodia/news/reaching-cambodias-last-mile-inclusive-and-sustainable-energy-access).

Clean water and sanitation coverage now reach 85% of the rural population. (Khmer Times, 21 March 2024, *Water supply, sanitation coverage in rural Cambodia hits 85 percent,* PM. Retrieved from https://www.khmertimeskh.com/501459775/water-supply-sanitation-coverage-in-rural-cambodia-hits-85-percent-)

Page 164: UNICEF said improving girl's education, particularly at the secondary level, leads to national growth, declining maternity mortality and child mortality rates, with less child stunting. (UNICEF, undated, *Girls' education, Gender equality in education benefits every child.* Retrieved www. unicef.org/education/girls-education).

Page 164: Thirty new schools were built, teachers training upgraded and over 400 school management committees formed, with community representatives. (World Bank, 16 August 2023, *Reforms Improve Education quality benefitting half a million students in Cambodia,* Retrieved https://www.worldbank.org/en/results/2023/08/16/reforms-improve-education-quality-benefitting-half-a-million-students-in-cambodia.)

Of those pregnant women who were HIV positive, over 32 percent received treatment, up from 11.2 percent in 2007. (UNAIDS, 20 September 2010, *Cambodia takes MDG prize for excellence in its AIDS response.* Retrieved from www.unaids.org/en/resources/presscentre/featurestories/2010/september/20100920fsmdgcamboda-award.)

However almost one quarter 23% of new infections were in Asia and the Pacific. (UNAIDS 2023, *The Path that ends AIDS, 2023 Global update,* Retrieved https://thepath.unaids.org/)

Pages 164-165: An estimated 86% of people living with HIV knew their status, with about 11,000 infected people remaining unaware of it. For people with HIV who were diagnosed 99% were on treatment and 98% had achieved viral suppression. (United Nations Cambodia, 5th April 2023, *Despite impressive treatment results Cambodia's HIV response must address inequalities affecting children and young key populations.* Retrieved from https://cambodia.un.org/en/226998-despite-impressive-treatment-results-cambodia%E2%80%99s-hiv-response-must-address-inequalities

List of Names

A   Arlys Herem, American Nurse who worked in the Thai border camps and then established an NGO, Dhammayietra, in Mongol Borei, Banteay Meanchey.

B   Bob Maat , Jesuit Brother, who worked in the border camps as a health worker, cofounded the national peace march, Dhammayietra, and lived and worked with the monks in Battambang at Wat Norea.

C   Corinne, Director of ZOA, a Dutch NGO based in Poipet.

D   Dyna, sex worker Phnom Penh, Member of Cambodian Prostitutes Association

E   Eap also known as Sin Eap, with Sin being his family name, Director of the Banteay Meanchey AIDS Officer and the author's counterpart.

G   Geoff Manthey, UNAIDS Director, Cambodia

Graham Forde, an Australian anthropologist who before arriving in Cambodia in 2001, worked in Thailand for many years.

M   Muny Vansaveth (Venerable) Head Monk Wat Norea, Peaceful Children.

Maha Gosandanda, Monk and founder with Bob Maat of monk's annual peace march, Dhammayietra, in Cambodia.

R   Renata Ran   UNAIDS Director South Pacific 2021.

S Sue McGlinchey (Authors deceased sister)

   Sin Eap (see Eap)

   Sarin Cambodian midwife, nurse and friend who worked with author.

   Sopheak Sarin's niece who following training worked with author.

   Sopheap Former monk and Religious Affairs officer at CARERE.

T Tia Phalla, Dr, Secretary General of the National AIDS Authority, Cambodia.

   Tess Experienced Thai Nurse who worked with Family Health International in Poipet.

   Tia Founder of the Cambodian Prostitutes Union.

Acronyms

ADB	Asian Development Bank
ADHOC	Cambodian Human Rights and Development Association
AEM	Asian Epidemic Model
AIDS	Acquired Immunodeficiency Syndrome
ANC	Antenatal Care
ART	Anti-retroviral therapy
ASEAN	Association of Southeast Asian Nations
AusAID	Australian Agency for International Development
AVI	Australian Volunteers International
BSS	Behavioural Surveillance Survey
CARE	International NGO worked with garment factory workers, motorcycle taxi drivers
CARERE	Cambodia Area Rehabilitation and Regeneration
CBO	Community-based organisation
CDC	Centre for Disease Control and Prevention
CMAC	Cambodian Mine Action Centre (Agency of Cambodian Government)
CoC	Continuum of Care
CRC	Cambodian Red Cross
100% CUP	100% Condom Use Program
CWCC	Cambodian Women's Crisis Centre

CWDA	Cambodian Women's Development Association
DAC	District AIDS Committee
DG	District Governor
DHS	Demographic and Health Survey
DOTS	Directly Observed Treatment, Short Course
DSW	Direct sex workers
ED	Essential Drug
EPI	Expanded Programme of Immunisation
EU	European Union
EW	Entertainment Workers
FGD	Focus Group Discussion
FHI	Family Health International
GAVI	Global Alliance for Vaccines and Immunisation
GBV	Gender Based Violence
GDP	Gross Domestic Product
GF	Global Fund
GFATM	Global Fund to Fight AIDS, Tuberculosis and Malaria
HAART	Highly Active Antiretroviral Therapy
HACC	HIV/AIDS Coordination Committee
HALO	Hazardous Area Life-support Organisation (demining)
HBC	Home-based care
HC	Health Centre
HEF	Health Equity Fund
HIS	Health Information System
HIV	Human Immunodeficiency Virus
HNI	HealthNet International

HSS	HIV Surveillance Study
IDUs	Injecting Drug Users
IDA	Iron Deficiency Anemia
IEC	Information, education, communication
IDSW	Indirect sex workers
JICA	Japan International Cooperation Agency
KAP	Knowledge, Attitudes and Practices
KHANA	Khmer HIV/AIDS NGO Alliance
M&E	Monitoring and Evaluation
MDG	Millennium Development Goals
MoCR	Ministry of Cults and Religion
MoEYS	Ministry of Education, Youth and Sport
MoH	Ministry of Health
MoND	Ministry of National Defence
MoSVY	Ministry of Social Affairs, Veterans, and Youth Rehabilitation
MoWA	Ministry of Women's Affairs
MoRD	Ministry of Rural Development
Motordops	Motorcycle taxi drivers
MSF	Medecins sans Frontieres
MSIC	Marie Stopes International Cambodia
MSM	Men who have sex with men
NAA	National AIDS Authority
NACD	National Authority for Combating Drugs
NBTC	National Blood Transfusion Centre
NCHADS	National Centre for HIV/AIDS, Dermatology & STI
NGO	Non-government organisations

NIS	National Institute of Statistics
NPA	Norwegian People's Aid
NSP	Needle and Syringe Program
OD	Operational District
OT	Opportunistic infections
OVC	Orphans and vulnerable children
Oxfam HK	Young women in the sex industry
PAO	Provincial AIDS Office
PAS	Provincial AIDS Secretariate
PATH	Program for Appropriate Technology in Health
PCP	Pneumocystis Pneumonia previously known as Pneumocystis Carinii
PE	Peer Educator
PEPFAR	President's Emergency Plan for AIDS Relief
PHD	Provincial Health Department
PLHA	People living with AIDS
PMTCT	Prevention of Mother to Child Prevention
PPH	Postpartum Hemorrhage
Pre-ART/ART	Pre-antiretroviral therapy/antiretroviral therapy
PSF	Pharmaciens Sans Frontieres
PSI	Population Service International
PWID	People who inject drugs
PWUD	People who use drugs
SEILA	Khmer for foundation
STI	Sexually transmitted Infections
TA	Technical Assistance
TB	tuberculosis

TBA	Traditional Birth Attendant
TH	Traditional Healer
Treatnet	International Network of treatment and rehabilitation treatment centres
TT	Tetanus toxoid
UNAIDS	Joint United Nations Program on HIV/AIDS
UNDP	United Nations Development Program
US CDC	United States Centres for Disease Control
UNESCO	United Nations Educational, Scientific and Cultural Organisation
UNFPA	United Nations Fund for Population Activities
UNICEF	United Nations Children's Fund
UNHCR	United Nations High Commissioner for Refugees
UNODC	United Nations Office on Drugs and Crime
UNTAC	United Nations Transitional Authority in Cambodia
USAID	United States Agency for International Development
VC	Village Chief
VCCT	Voluntary and confidential counselling and testing
VHV	Village health volunteer
VTC	Voluntary Testing Centre
WAD	World AIDS Day
WATSAN	Water and Sanitation
WFP	World Food Program
WHO	World Health Organisation

WVC	World Vision Cambodia
YSRH	Youth Sexual Reproductive Health
ZOA	Dutch NGO. ZOA stands for South East Asia in Dutch

www.ingramcontent.com/pod-product-compliance
Lightning Source LLC
LaVergne TN
LVHW011910080426
835508LV00007BA/331